CRISIS PREVENTION & INTERVENTION

IN HEALTHCARE

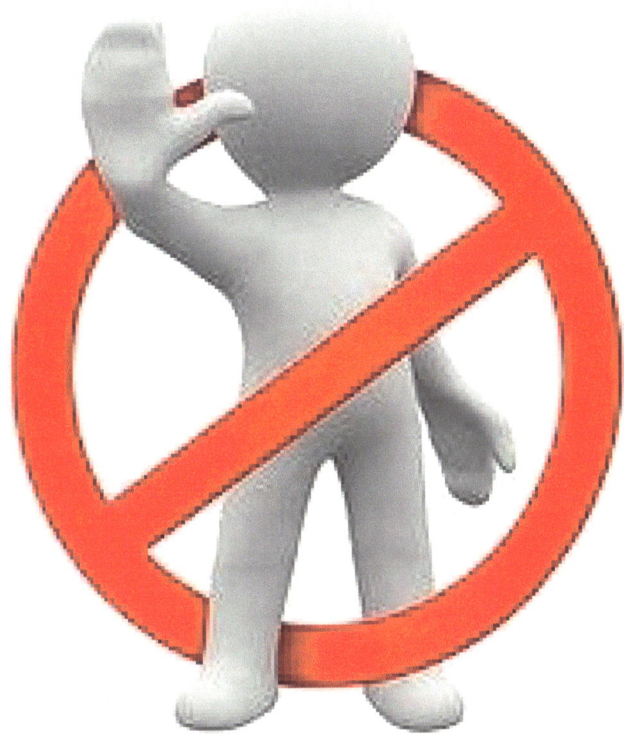

ACPMA

AMERICAN CRISIS PREVENTION & MANAGEMENT ASSOCIATION

RIGHT KNOWLEDGE, RIGHT RESPONSE

Crisis Prevention & Intervention

In Healthcare

ISBN-13: 978-0988911727

ISBN-10: 0988911728

Printed in the United States of America.

www.acpmaonline.com
www.americancrisispreventionandmanagementassociation.com

Acknowledgement

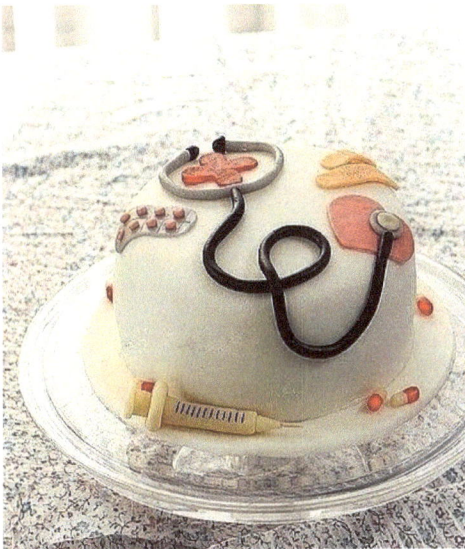

To all the nurses, doctors and administrative staff that contributed to the success of this publication, thank you!

About ACPMA

The American Crisis Prevention and Management Association (ACPMA) has been providing crisis prevention, intervention and management training and consulting for many years. ACPMA trainers are experienced crisis prevention and management consultants that bring the knowledge needed to help individuals and organizations excel. Our organizational board consists of nurses and doctors who in addition to their wealth of experience, conduct continuous research towards reducing the problems arising from behavioral crisis.

Table of Contents

Preface

Introduction

Chapter 1
Meaning of Crisis, types and causes

Chapter 2
General safety measures, personal safety

Chapter 3
The assault cycle, violent predictive behaviors

Chapter 4
Obtaining history, Characteristics of violent patients & victims.

Chapter 5
Verbal & physical maneuvers to diffuse & avoid physical harm

Chapter 6
Restraining techniques, use of medication

Chapter 7
Emergency Preparedness by Hospitals

Preface

How can you respond to a situation when you do not know what to do? That is why we believe that the *right knowledge* leads to the *right response*

-ACPMA

Introduction

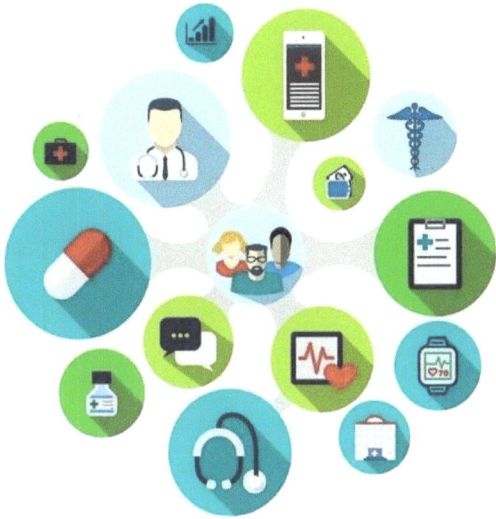

The purpose of this book is to ensure that strategies are employed as early as possible in a situation to detect aggressive factors early, prevent escalation of emotions that could result in assaultive behavior and crisis, and to know the right intervention in case it takes place. Strength is given to the old saying "Prevention is better than cure".

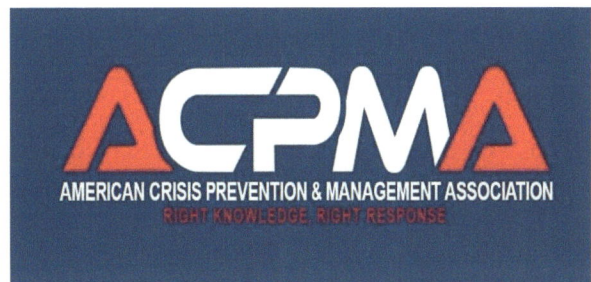

CHAPTER ONE

<u>OUTLINE</u>

1.0 Introduction

2.0 Meaning of Crisis

2.1 Definitions

2.2 Background of Crisis

2.3 Features of crisis

2.4 Examples of Crisis

2.5 Corresponding factors of assaultive behavior/crisis

3.0 Types of crisis and their causes

3.1 Criminal crisis

3.2 Patient crisis

3.3 Worker crisis

3.4 Domestic crisis

3.5 Verbal and physical crisis

4.0 Conclusion

Crisis Prevention and Intervention in Healthcare

1.0 INTRODUCTION

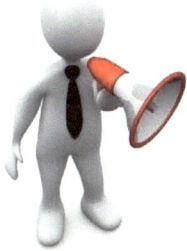

The management of assaultive behavior is intended to provide protection for the client and healthcare professional against any type of assault from either party. Assaultive behavior in the healthcare setting compromises the safety of the healthcare workers, the patients and visitors to the emergency rooms, mental health units, group homes, long term care facilities, etc.

The abusive behavior undermines the efforts of the health care professionals that are in many cases, the victims. Poor behavior management costs the hospital time, money and high turnover rates. This chapter will discuss the meaning of assaultive behavior and crisis, as well as discuss the types and causes of crisis.

2.0 WHAT IS CRISIS?

2.1 Definitions

The meaning of crisis can be expanded by defining crisis, assaultive behavior and violence. According to Aguilera (1998, p. 12), crisis occurs when a person is unable to deal with problems that seem not to have a way out. The unresolved problems give way to anger, emotional unrest, tension, anxiety and stagnation.

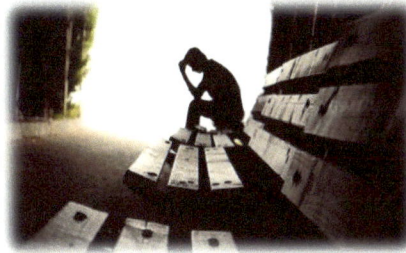

- Crisis is viewed as a psychological instability that result from extreme situation or condition where the resolution is not attainable by means of common remedies.

- Crisis can also be used to define to a situation where assaultive behavior or violence has occurred. Great emphasis is placed on ensuring that strategies are employed as early as possible in the process to detect potential situations early, prevent escalation of emotions that could result in assaultive behavior and effectively manage the crisis situation if it occurs.

Crisis is used to refer to assaultive behavior when it is extremely negative, unpredictable, uncontrollable and unacceptable in the society.

2.2   Background of Crisis

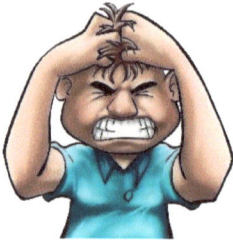

Assaultive behavior can occur anywhere and the hospital or other healthcare settings are not exceptions.

People without any history of assaultive behavior or psychiatric condition can suddenly become combative.

➢ Assaultive behavior can be as a result of medical conditions or illnesses as well as certain medications.

➢ Assaultive behavior is present in people of all cultures, and socio-economic status. Crisis may also be as a result of unresolved emotional issues.

➢ People experiencing crisis desire to solve the problem as quickly as possible. They are influenced by actions or words from others, because they crave for a solution that can change their situation.

Assaultive behavior may be directed to:

+ Relatives or family members
+ Neighbors
+ Roommates
+ Authority figures
+ Men
+ Women
+ Medical professionals
+ Peers
+ Bystanders and
+ Passive peers.

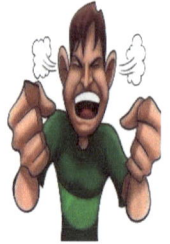

The assault can be done in the home, care facility, homeless shelter, hospital, school or correctional institutions.

The common assaults involve the use of a

1. Weapon,

2. Physical violence and

3. Throwing of objects.

The medical conditions that have been found capable of leading to assaultive behavior include:

1. Vascular dementia

2. Alzheimer's

3. Diabetes

4. Stroke

5. Delirium

6. Excessive alcohol and

7. Medicine intoxication.

Features of Crisis

1 Crisis that involves assaultive behavior or violence poses a threat.

2 The crisis reveals a persistent inability to change condition or eliminate the effects of the underlying issues.

3 Crisis invites tension, confusion and fear.

4 The person in crisis experiences a lot of discomfort.

5 The person in crisis remains in a disequilibrium state.

6 Crisis can be said to be forthcoming if the client has a record of violent behavior and tendencies of verbal abuse towards others.

2.3 Examples of Crisis

Crisis occurs when a person is physically sick or a close person is sick.

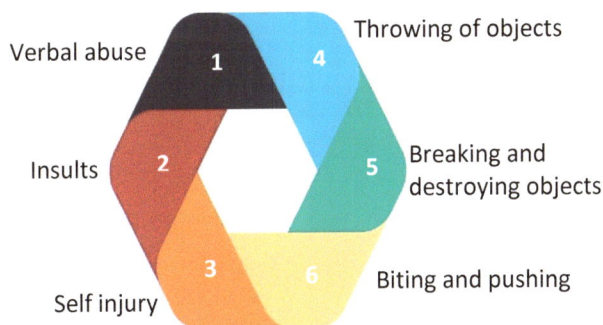

Other examples of crisis include: divorce or separation, loss of a person through death, accident, natural calamity, financial constraints, unwanted pregnancy and unemployment. If there is no intervention to the underlying situation , it may lead to trauma.

2.4 Corresponding factors of Assaultive behavior/ Crisis

In an attempt to understand the meaning of crisis, Aguilera (1998, p. 13) discussed three corresponding factors that a person with assaultive behavior experiences. The corresponding factors involves:

- **PERCEPTION**
- **SUPPORT**
- **SURVIVAL**

Perception deals with the attitude and view the person with assaultive behavior has towards the underlying problem. The underlying problem could be finances, health, reputation, work, education and career which are very important to the person.

In a mental health patient, the individual has the paranoia that the nurses have bad plans against him. That is why, when there are a group of people around them, they need proper explanation as to why they are in the midst of a crowd.

If a good explanation is not proffered and on time, they may perceive themselves as 'trapped' and start violent actions like attacking anybody in the group or throwing objects.

Healthcare professionals must remember that mental health patients have auditory hallucinations which they feel compelled to obey.

3.0 TYPES OF CRISIS AND THEIR CAUSES

According to Colling and York (2010, p. 484) crisis can be distinguished according to the person who performs the assault and event.

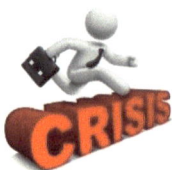

The four types of crisis include;

1. Criminal,
2. Patient,
3. Worker and
4. Domestic.

3.1 Criminal Crisis / Assaultive Behavior.

The individual performing the assault may not be related to the healthcare institution or the patient.

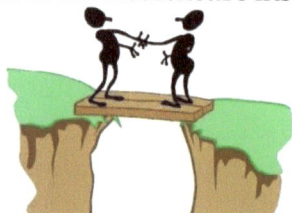

This can be a criminal who finds his way into the healthcare facility. They may rob or steal items belonging to patients, visitors or the health care facility. Criminal crisis happens because of availability of weapons such as guns.

When the hospital security is weak, the criminals may find the hospital accessible and commit crimes. The hospital may lack movement restrictions within the medical facility.

Because of the existence of safes in the hospital where patients' money, jewelry and other valuable items are stored, it could become a target for robbery. Some criminals choose to abduct patients receiving treatment and become violent when committing the act. Criminals causing problems in healthcare facilities consist of terrorists and unwanted visitors. The criminals may pose as legitimate visitors to the patient or as health care workers (Salmon and Varela, 2007, p. 4).

3.2 Patient Crisis

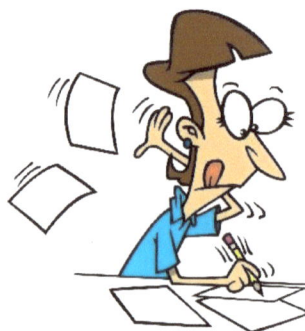

The patient receiving healthcare service can become aggressive. Patient crisis is caused by patients who are receiving treatment. Some of the patients may be mentally disturbed and cause harm to others. Some patients who are mentally ill, abuse drugs, are traumatized or are frustrated by the situations; hence they become aggressive.

The patient may take advantage of a situation where the healthcare worker is alone in the health care facility, possibly performing a medical examination in an isolated room without the company of another person.

They may use their nails, fists, body fluids, feet, teeth, food utensils, head, furniture or medical equipment to inflict injury on the healthcare professional (Charney and Fragala 2000, p. 163).

3.3 Worker Crisis

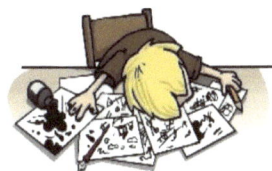

Worker crisis involves a healthcare professional of the healthcare facility. The aggression may be directed towards another worker, patient or a visitor. Healthcare workers may have underlying disputes with each other that could result in aggressiveness.

Depending on the nature of their dispute and anger management, the unresolved conflict may result in violence. The employees may work within the same department and rank at the same level.

The common forms of abuse can be overt or covert. Overt abuse can be in the form of verbal abuse. Covert abuse takes the form of psychological harassment.

The uncomfortable situation may be motivated by the workers withholding information from each other, change of duties without consenting and informing the other, criticism, isolation and refusing to assist at work (Richter and Whittington 2006, p. 3).

A typical example is a nurse who always comes late. Everybody on the unit knows that if they are assigned to relieve someone, the outgoing nurse would never leave on time. Such behaviors can result in unpleasant open confrontations and arguments on the medical unit.

Lannza (2006, p. 86) adds that, the health care provider may experience stress because of understaffing and workload.

3.4 Domestic Crisis

Domestic violence can be said to occur in the healthcare institution where the patient, the health care worker, relatives and friends to the patient engage in assaultive behavior.

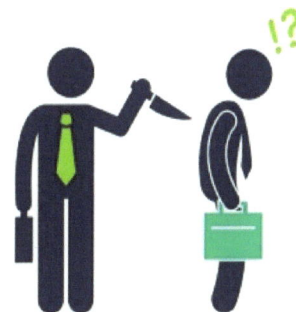

The relatives and friend to the patient may become impatient if the hospital takes long to attend to the patient, delays treatment or medical procedures. On another note, the relatives or friends may have personal differences with the patient and resolve them in the hospital.

An example could be an abusive husband whom the wife is hospitalized as a result of his actions. He then meets face to face with the mother of the victim at the bedside.

Also, the patient's relatives could become assaultive because of experiencing stress that comes with the patient illness. An argument can quickly escalate into a fight because of financial, emotional and excessive anger that either the patient or their visitor may be experiencing.

3.5 Verbal and Physical Abuse

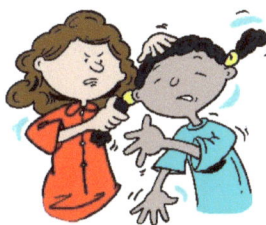

Physical abuse is directed to others, self and objects.

The patient, health care worker, visitor or criminal may become violent to another person and beat, bite, slap, hit or push them. The patient can hurt self by biting, cutting and inflicting injury on the body. In some cases, a patient, visitor, health care worker or criminal may throw objects towards another out of anger.

Whether verbally or physically assaultive, a patient can become uncomfortable in their environment and become irritable as Duxbury and Whittington (2005, p. 472) discuss. A restrictive environment can become a source of conflict.

Crisis can be caused by internal, external or interactional factors. The patient may have mental illness or be under the influence of medication that can cause aggression. The healthcare worker or the patient's visitor may also have internal perception of the issues concerned and become violent. Internal aspects of crisis involve thought disorders, alcohol abuse and substance abuse.

Crisis refers to assaultive behavior or violence that occurs after an individual is unable to change uncomfortable circumstances, becomes unpredictable, unmanageable and their behavior is not approved in the society. Crisis occurs when an individual cannot change circumstances and the available resources are limited.

4.0 CONCLUSION

Types of crisis/ assaultive behavior include: criminal, patient, worker and domestic crisis. People with crisis engage in physical and verbal abuse. Crisis is triggered by internal, external and situational factors. Medication, illness, substance abuse, lack of training for workers, unresolved emotional issues, lack of communication, long waiting time, delayed or denied services and poor security could lead to assaultive behavior.

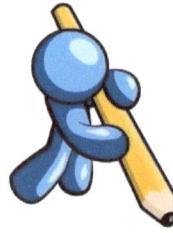

REFERENCES

Aguilera, D. C. (1998). *Crisis intervention: Theory and methodology* (8th ed.).

St. Louis: Mosby Charney, W., and Fragala, G. (2000). *The Epidemic of Health Care Worker Injury: An Epidemiology.* Florida: CRC Press.

Chou, K. R., Lu, R. B., and Chang, M. (2001). Assaultive behavior by psychiatric in-patient and its related factors. *Journal of Nursing Research,* 9 (15), 139- 151.

Colling, R. L., and York, T. W. (2010). *Hospital and healthcare security* (5th ed.). New York: Elsevier Inc.

Duxbury, J., and Whittington, R. (2005). Causes and management of patient aggression and violence: staff and patient perspectives *Journal of Advanced Nursing* 50(5), 469–478

Lannza, M. L., Zeiss, R and Rierdan, J. (2006). Violence against psychiatric nursing. *Contemporary Nurse,* 21(1), 85-93.

Quanbeck, C. D. (2007). Categorization of aggressive behavior acts committed by a chronically assaultive state hospital patient. *Psychiatric Services* 58 (4), 521- 528.

Richter, D., and Whittington, R. (2006). *Violence in Mental Health Settings: Causes, Consequences, Management,* Berlin: Springer.

Salmon, N., and Varela, R. (2007) *Learning to manage assaultive behavior.* New York: AMN Healthcare Services Inc.

Shaver, P. R., and Mikulincer, M. (2010) *Human Aggression and Violence: Causes, Manifestations, and Consequences.* Washington: American Psychological Association.

CHAPTER TWO

<u>OUTLINE</u>

1.0 Introduction

2.0 General Safety Measures for the Healthcare Professionals

2.1 Administration and healthcare professional support

2.2 Environmental analysis

2.3 Risk reduction

2.4 Training

2.5 Regular review

3.0 Personal Safety Measures

3.1 Education and Training

3.2 Self defense mechanisms

3.3 Ways of de-escalating violence

3.4 Be alert

3.5 Self-care for professional healthcare

4.0 Conclusion

Safety Measures to Prevent or Reduce Crisis in Healthcare

1.0 INTRODUCTION

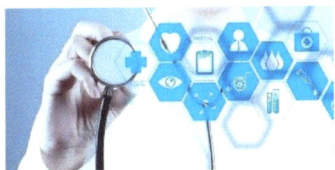

The management of assaultive behavior in healthcare facility involves promoting the safety of patients, healthcare professionals and visitors. This chapter will discuss general and personal safety measures in the healthcare facility.

2.0 GENERAL SAFETY MEASURES FOR THE HEALTHCARE PROFESSIONALS

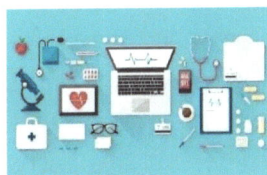

General safety measures for health care professionals facilitate sustenance of a good working environment and prevention of assaultive behavior. The safety measures should be adjusted according to specific conditions or nature of environment that healthcare professionals work in.

General safety measures consist of five elements;

1. Administration and Healthcare
2. Professional Support,
3. Environmental Analysis,
4. Risk reduction,
5. Training and Regular Review

2.1 Administration and Healthcare Professional Support

The healthcare administration and the facility employees must engage in safety plans. The plans involve appointing teams of healthcare workers, employers, committees and representatives of the safety plans. The healthcare professionals who are experts in crisis management should be involved. This can include the quality control department to set standards and the education department to train the employees.

The representation should be fair in terms of departments and shifts. Drills should be conducted for workers in the different shifts. i.e. drills should be conducted for the night shift workers, morning shift workers and mid-shift workers, so that everyone is equipped with knowledge of early recognition and appropriate intervention of assaultive behaviors.

Tasks should be allocated to the different stakeholders who may include:

+ Employer's representative,
+ Healthcare professionals,
+ Security representatives and Administrators.

Healthcare professionals able to deal with head injury, substance abuse, psychiatry and dementia should be advised to assist when the need arises. A working structure and applicable policies can be designed. The policies should represent diverse needs of the departments and provide procedures to be used in case of crisis.

The safety plan should take into consideration the physical, psychological and emotional safety and health of the healthcare professionals. A balance between the safety and health needs of the healthcare professional, patient or visitor should be recommended. Representatives, experts, committees and teams with assigned tasks or responsibility should inquire and understand their responsibility in full detail.

The healthcare professionals ought to be committed to comply with the policies and give feedback. Suggestions on safety and complains should be given the appropriate authority. Cases of crisis should be reported in time and appropriately, and affected individuals receive treatment per facility policies.

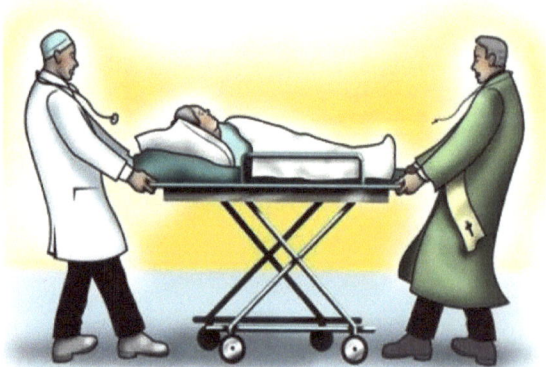

2.2 Environmental Analysis.

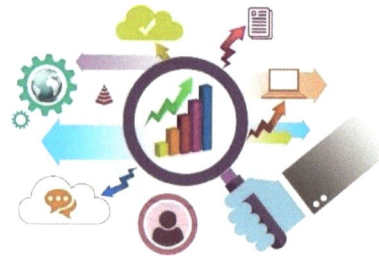

Environmental analysis will consist of an assessment where potential risks are identified. Procedures, threats and factors that could result in unwanted situations are pointed out. The analysis will take into consideration incidents and history of assaultive behavior in the same and other healthcare facilities. The information could be retrieved from compensation claims and patient records.

Environmental analysis in the workplace focuses on records, surveys and security details. The records will give details of occurrence of incidents in various departments, healthcare professionals by title, time, activities in progress and frequency of occurrence. The incidents are analyzed and compared with similar reports from other healthcare facilities. Surveys taken from healthcare professionals can be a source of information.

The surveys can assist in determining procedures that lead to risks, inadequate measures, inadequate resources, failures, policies and activities that need to be changed. Characteristics of those involved in the assaultive behavior and recommendations are considered.

Risky procedures and locations should be identified. Some of the factors may involve physical conditions like the layout of the hospital facility. Isolated locations, lack of communication, security problems and inadequate light that contribute to risk.

2.3   Risk Reduction

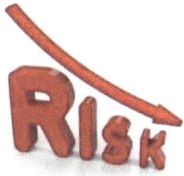

Risk can be reduced by adopting measures, procedures and administrative work that will assist in preventing and controlling the occurrence of assaultive behavior in the health facility.

The administration should make physical changes to the environment. The changes may consist of adequate lighting in dark rooms and increased space where necessary. There should be light both inside and outside the healthcare facility.

Alarm system and panic buttons can be installed so that a potential victim can obtain assistance. The phones and radio systems should be working at all times and reliable.

- The waiting room should be made comfortable with chairs and reading materials.
- The furniture should be placed properly to avoid falls.
- The number of furniture in the consultation room and activity room should be limited.
- The furniture should not be fixed or possess sharp ends.
- Avoid placing vases, pictures or trays where they are visible or in high risk areas.
- The healthcare professionals will require different washrooms from the patients installed with locks.
- Broken furniture, bulbs, windows and locks should be replaced.
- Thorough searching of mental health patients during admission must be done to prevent smuggling tiny weapons like razor blades, needles, tiny pocket knives, etc.
- Every pocket comb must be completely examined as some pocket combs, when unfolded are pocket knives.
- Patients must account for their tooth brushes as some mental health patients break their brushes and use them as weapons.

2.4 Training

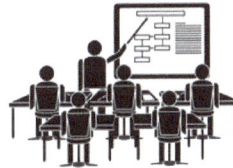

Mason and Chandley (1999, p. 65) educates that training provides understanding on assaultive behavior, and enables the healthcare professionals to prevent and handle impending crisis appropriately.

Training educates the healthcare professional on policies concerning assaultive behavior in the healthcare facility. Additionally, the healthcare professionals will be able to recognize risks, escalating behavior, warning signs, prevention methods and what to do in the case of a crisis. They will know where to report and how to report an unpleasant incident.

Additional information about cultural diversity, personality differences and various ailments that contribute to assaultive behavior can be shared (Flannery 1998, p. 91). They will also know how to complain or itemize concerns, where to complain and how to get compensation. Training should be given to healthcare professionals, managers, supervisors, security workers, and other hospital workers.

2.5 Regular Review

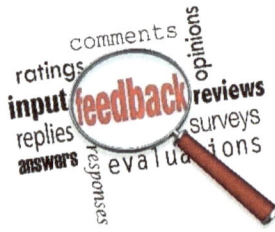

Records of assaultive behavior should be made. Most facilities call it the incident report. The records should be analyzed to give information on risk factors and patterns of assault. An analysis will provide a basis for identifying gaps that can be made to manage assaultive behavior in the healthcare facility.

Important items for record include: type of injury, number of incidents, assault, threat, accidents, type of crisis, response to crisis, persons involved, identified problem and solutions.

3.0 PERSONAL SAFETY MEASURES

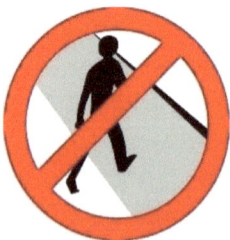

Healthcare professionals should assume responsibility for their individual safety. They need to protect self from possible aggressive behavior coming from patients, visitors and other healthcare professionals. This can be achieved through: education and training which is the reason for this textbook, self defense mechanisms, de-escalating violence, being alert and practicing extreme environmental awareness.

Healthcare workers should take their breaks in protected rooms that the patients do not have access to.

There was a case of a nurse on duty who was supposed to be watching a patient on a one-to-one observation to prevent suicide. Unfortunately, the nurse slept off, the patient beat the nurse so bad that by the time, the other workers could arrive, she was already unconscious. She was rushed to the emergency room and suffered paralysis from spinal cord injury inflicted by the patient.

3.1 Education and Training

As healthcare professionals engage in ongoing training, the employee will assist in raising the awareness of the trigger factors.

Employees will understand safety strategies and techniques for conducting self at work. Training will educate the healthcare professionals on the techniques for de-escalating violence.

Bibby (1995, p. 56) found out that, education gives the healthcare professional the ability to predict behavior and adjust to being neutral in the diffusion of anger.

The healthcare professionals should cooperate with the organization when asked to join in programs. The policies concerning the working environment should be followed. All incidents should be reported to the appropriate authority so that appropriate measures are taken to prevent further assaultive incidents. The healthcare facility puts a lot of effort in the prevention and management of crisis.

3.2   Self defense Mechanisms

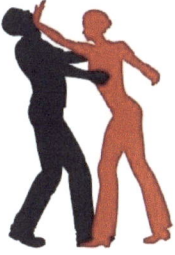

A professional healthcare worker can practice safety by adapting appropriated behavior and choosing to defend self in the case of a physical assault.

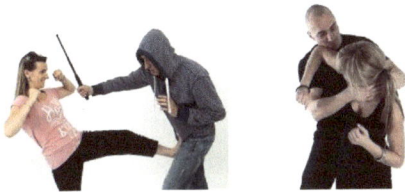

When at risk, they can call for assistance, keep the way clear and escape if possible.

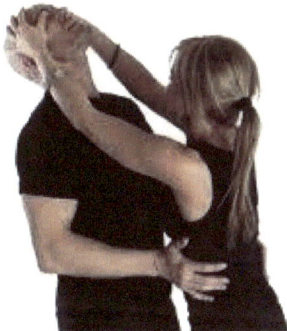

Practice patience and encourage conversation. Avoid showing the aggressive person the back, as the aggressor can try to choke from the back and get away.

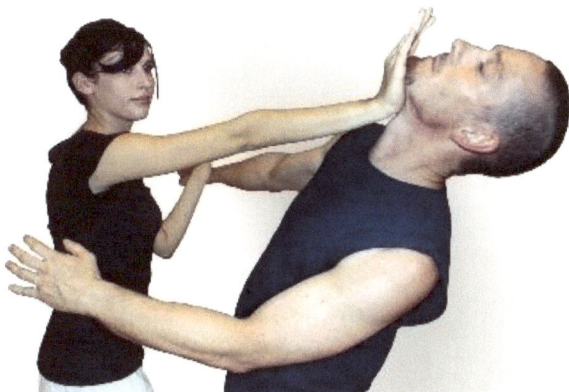

Another way of protecting self is by choking the aggressor from the front if they attack from the front. If the attacker grabs the arm, try to push the arms downwards then twist towards the escape route.

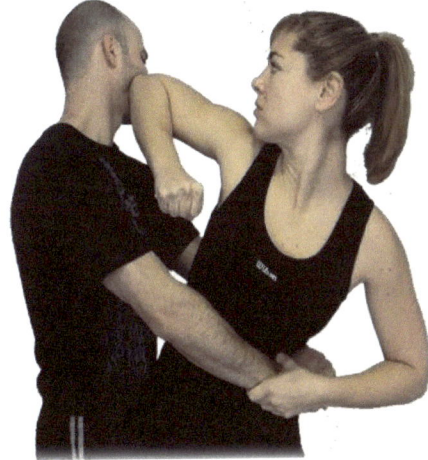

Personal safety measures require a healthcare professional to avoid working in isolation where there are patients with assaultive behavior.

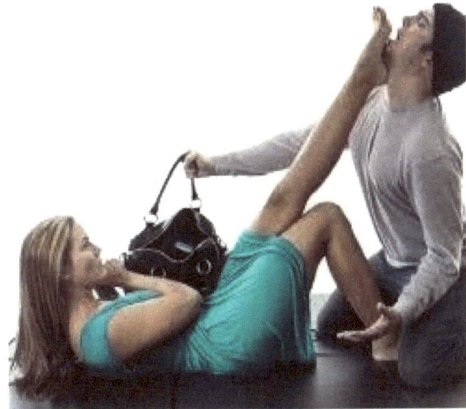

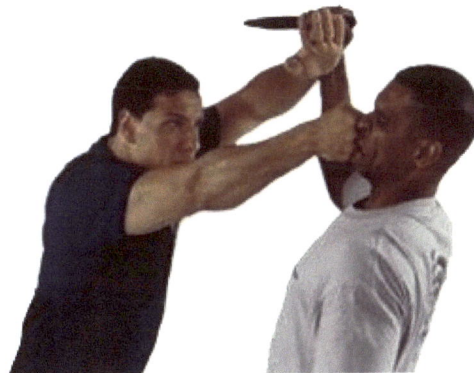

3.3   Ways of De-escalating Violence

For personal protection, a healthcare professional can bargain and apply conflict resolution when facing a possible crisis. Conversations should be conducted in a calm environment with the worker listening to the person in crisis.

Confrontation should be avoided, keep away from persistent contact of the eyes. It is wise to stay away from interacting and request for audience. Showing empathy, understanding and showing concern to the assaultive person can reduce tension. Healthcare professionals can use moderate tone, calm voice and appropriate choice of words when communicating. Redirecting the topic can be another significant method of de-escalating assaultive behavior.

Refrain from responding to threats with other threats since it can activate violence.

An example is an incident where a mental health patient told a nurse that she should be ashamed of herself because all she does is come to the hospital to give meds to make a living.

The nurse replied her that she should be more ashamed that her teenage mates are in college, working, or at least doing something with their lives, but she is 'living' in the hospital. The patient reacted in a way that was very notable. There was a code gray.

When the root of the behavior was researched, the nurse gave the story. Avoid commanding and when given a chance acknowledge their feelings. Evade walking close, jumping, touching or moving closely to the person with signs of aggression. Avoid touching objects that could be perceived as a weapon.

Communicate when you want to move or touch them by making them understand your purpose. The healthcare professional can request for permission before dressing a wound, changing beddings, taking temperature or recording blood pressure, when conducting medical procedures (Scott et al 2001, p. 61).

3.4   Be Alert

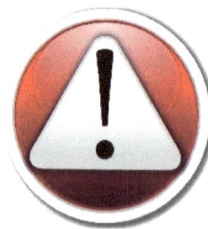

The healthcare professional should be very alert, taking precaution when a threat of aggressiveness is imminent. They should enact a safety plan without delay if a patient is assaultive. If the healthcare professionals are threatened, they should avoid using suggestive body language and words that may reveal their feelings to the patient.

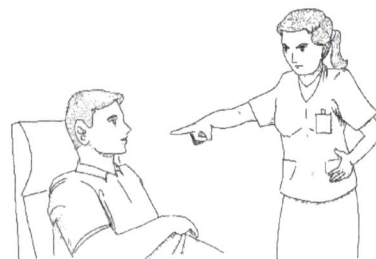

If the patients detect a threat, they may withhold information, feel threatened and react negatively to the healthcare provider's instructions (Hamilton 2011, p. 1).

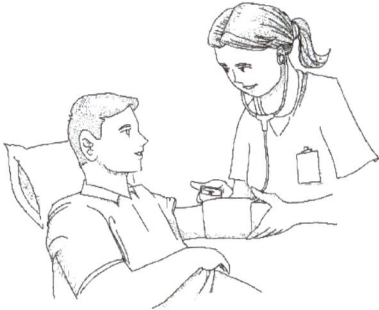

According to Hughes (2008, p. 39), the healthcare professionals should be able to recognize risks and signs that can lead to aggressive behavior. Nurses and other healthcare workers should recognize signs of assaultive behavior. When a person shows frustration, anger and physical gestures depicting aggression, they can be viewed as a threat.

- ❖ Recognize patients with conditions that cause aggression such as mental illness and head injury.
- ❖ Remain alert at all times because every situation is unique and should be handled depending on the circumstances.
- ❖ Healthcare professionals should analyze the situation and type of occurrence before attending to the patient.
- ❖ Exercise vigilance when dealing with the patient.

3.5 Self-care for Healthcare Professional

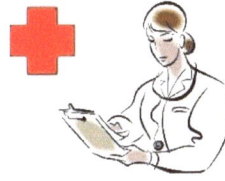

Healthcare professionals may become busy and fail to take care of their needs which can contribute to emotional outbursts. With the knowledge of their working environment and challenges, healthcare workers should take care of their emotional, physical and psychological needs. The healthcare professionals should regulate the number of hours in a day so that they are not overworked.

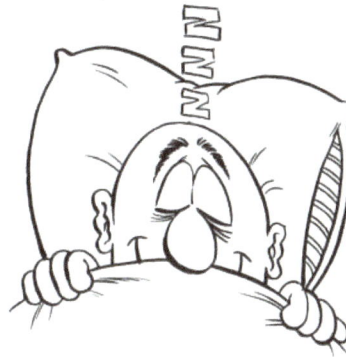

After work they should rest and get enough sleep. It is very ironical how healthcare professionals preach so much about rest but rarely observe it. They are many a time ruled by the amount of money they will make when they work overtimes. Lack of time for oneself can predispose to lack of mental alertness when assaultive behavior is imminent.

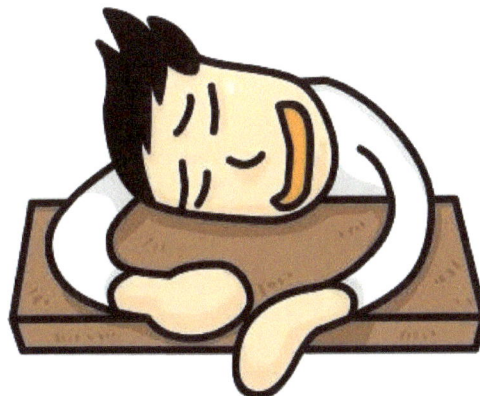

Evade situation that can cause burnout and fatigue. Healthcare professionals can manage stress by performing hypnosis techniques. The healthcare professionals should take a balanced diet and have regular physical exercises. They can maintain social relations with family and friends for social support.

Healthcare professionals should maintain their spiritual relations and stay proactive (National Collaborating Centre for Nursing and Supportive Care, 2005 p. 1).

General safety measures require improvement of the physical environment, improved working relations with patients and other healthcare employees, participation in implementation plan and reporting incidents correctly to the right authorities.

Personal safety measures encourage healthcare professionals to ensure they receive training and competence in assaultive behavior prevention and management.

4.0 CONCLUSION

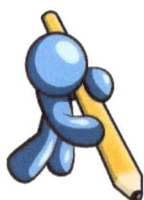

General and personal safety measures facilitate prevention and intervention of aggressive behavior. Healthcare facility administration and healthcare professionals are required to collaborate in the development plan of policies and intervention of violent behavior. After developing a plan, the selected teams, commissioners and representatives analyze the environment to identify the risk factors.

The healthcare facility together with professionals commit themselves to strategies that help in reducing risks that could contribute to crisis. Healthcare employees are trained on the safety measures, warning signs and intervention. Once the plans are implemented, they are reviewed regularly and adjusted accordingly.

REFERENCE

Bartholomew, K. (2006). *Ending Nurse-To-Nurse Hostility Why Nurses Eat Their Young and Each Other.* Danvers: HCPro.

Bibby, P. (1995). *Personal Safety for Health Care Workers (Suzy Lamplugh Trust)*

Farnham: Ashgate Publishing Limited. Flannery, R. (1998). *Violence in the Workplace Managing Assaultive Behavior.* New York: Crossroad publishing company.

Hamilton, P. M. (2011). *Psychiatric Emergencies: Caring for People in Crisis.* Wild Iris Medical Education Inc.

Hughes, R. (2008). Patient safety and quality: an evidence based Handbook for nurses. Agency for Healthcare Research & Quality.

Linsley, P. (2006). *Violence and Aggression in the Workplace: A Practical Guide for All Healthcare Staff.* Abingdon: Radcliffe Publishing.

Mason T & Chandley M. (1999). *Management of violence and aggression.* Philadelphia: Churchill Livingstone.

National Collaborating Centre for Nursing and Supportive Care. (2005) VIOLENCE: THE SHORT-TERM MANAGEMENT OF DISTURBED/ VIOLENT BEHAVIOUR IN PSYCHIATRIC IN-PATIENT SETTINGS AND EMERGENCY DEPARTMENTS. London: National Institute for Clinical Excellence.

Occupational Safety and Health Administration (2011). *Guidelines for Preventing Workplace Violence for Health Care & Social Service Workers.* United States: U.S. Department of Labor.

Scott, S., Chris, W., and Sorensen, S. (2001) Essentials of aggression management in health care. New Jersey: Prentice Hall.

CHAPTER THREE

<u>OUTLINE</u>

1.0 Introduction

2.0 The Assault Cycle

2.1 Trigger phase

2.2 Escalation phase

2.3 Crisis phase

2.4 Recovery phase

2.5 Post crisis phase

3.0 Aggression and Violent Predictive Factors

3.1 Demography and personal history

3.2 Individual disorders, sickness and substance abuse factors

3.3 Situational factors

3.4 Actuarial and clinical predictive factors

3.5 Broset violence register

4.0 Conclusion

Crisis Prevention and Intervention in Healthcare

1.0 INTRODUCTION

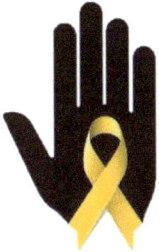

A clear pattern of how violence occurs has been identified. There are preceding observations that can be made before a person progresses to become assaultive (Linsley, 2000, p. 48). This chapter will describe the cycle of assaultive behavior, provide predictive factors for aggression and violence and educate on the appropriate interventions.

2.0 THE ASSAULT CYCLE

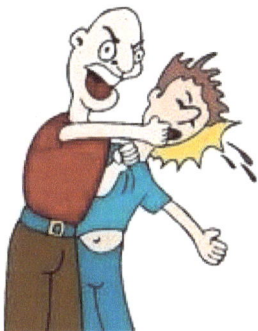

The assault cycle has distinct patterns that can assist in predicting violence and enable the health care professional to administer appropriate measures. The patterns in assaultive behavior are common in different groups, genders and persons. In every cycle, different behaviors can be observed in particular phases.

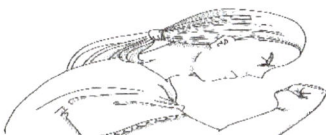

The five phases of the assault cycle include:

1. Trigger,
2. Escalation,
3. Crisis,
4. Recovery
5. Post crisis.

2.1. Trigger Phase

An individual begins to detect threats to their security or welfare. Feelings of being denied, being ignored or being refused something important to them crop in. The aggressor then becomes frustrated as Linsley (2006, p. 48) highlights.

A person in trigger phase perceives that they have lost control. They review the issues facing them and see the magnitude of the conflict as huge. Fear is real and the person in crisis tries to compensate for what they are denied. They may be in denial and reason with self to justify events.

The trigger is as a result of other people's actions, an argument with another person, upsetting information an in- ability to do something they have been denied such as consuming alcohol or even a smoke break. Crisis can be eliminated if the problems and conflicts are solved. Trigger phase is not associated with experiences of medication or hallucinations.

The appropriate response towards the potentially aggressive person would be to divert their mind and engage them in a meaningful discussion. Exercising good communication skills where one remains neutral would be helpful. The therapeutic communication skills used in this intervention is called **verbal de-escalation**. Discuss the issue making the patient uncomfortable and try to proffer solution.

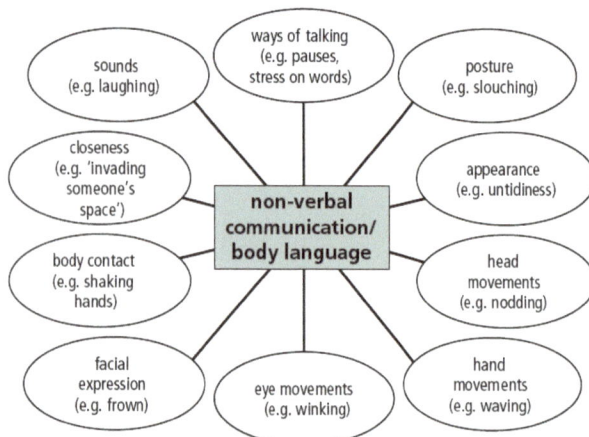

A healthcare professional can alert others and record observations. The healthcare professional should remain calm and avoid showing signs of fear. Keep a distance, show the hands and stay close to exit.

2.2. Escalation Phase

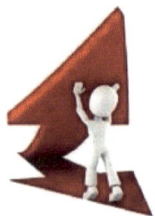

The assaultive person begins to prepare for aggression. Threats are presented verbally to the prospective victim if they are within reach.

Anger steps in and the aggressor throws objects, begins pacing and kicking walls. The voice is raised and yelling that is sometimes accompanied by banging is experienced or seen.

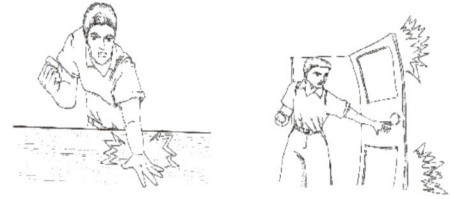

The escalating phase provides an opportunity for a healthcare professional trained in crisis intervention to employ de-escalating techniques to prevent violence from occurring. If possible, explaining to the aggressive person that consequences of violence can be severe can be helpful. This can be done with caution because it can be perceived as a threat to the aggressor.

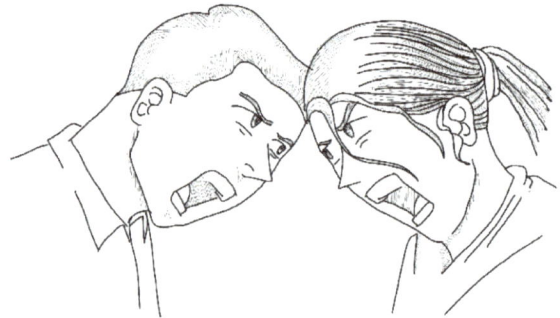

Adamowski et al (2009, p. 740) adds that, the thinking process is affected by the high levels of anger and distress. Consequently, the aggressor begins to become dysfunctional, disorganized and lacks sleep. They may direct their anger to animals or objects rather than directing them towards a person. Very minor events become a cause of argument.

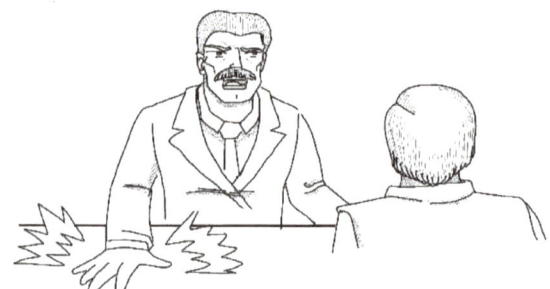

2.3. Crisis Phase

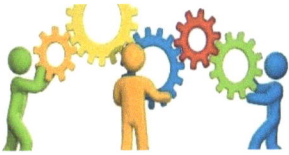

Crisis stage involves actual aggressive behavior. The aggressor assaults the seeming threat. A lot of energy is used in violence. The assaultive individual becomes weary very quick because the energy to sustain an attack is limited.

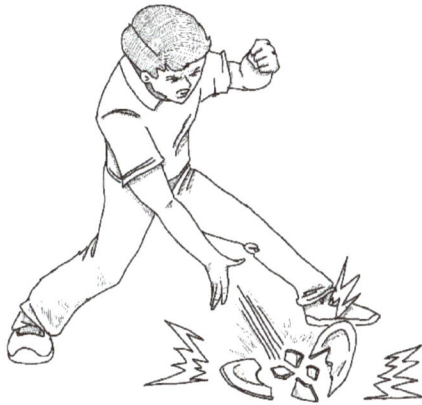

In the crisis phase, the aggressor dominates the victim by controlling with violence. The abuser is unpredictable and fears losing power, therefore, they use violence to control. The aggressor believes it is the victim on the wrong. The victim of assaultive behavior is abused, feels helpless and becomes traumatized.

To ensure they have control, the abuser takes time to decide words to use and place they will use for abuse. They scheme and attempt to do what they have planned on the victim.

2.4. Recovery Phase

After becoming assaultive, the aggressor slows down to recover. The aggressor is watchful and any impending threats could generate another assault.

The feeling of being disorganized remains and the aggressor becomes confused.

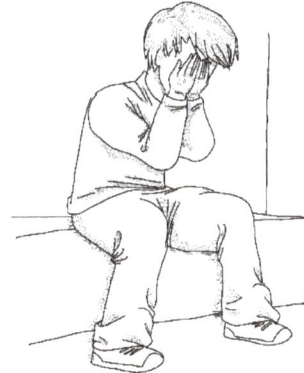

In the attempt to recover what has been damaged, the aggressor reconciles by showing affection and apologizing. The abuser ends violence and demonstrates their desire to change. Because of feeling remorseful the aggressor becomes sad and shows that they are repentant.

In some cases the aggressor refuses to apologize and ignores the violent event. They leave the victim without saying a word and disappear. Some return and request the victim to sympathize with them. They become very convincing to justify their act and profess that they will not repeat assault.

2.5. Post Crisis Phase

The aggressive individual calms down and becomes emotional about their actions. They show intense remorse, fatigue and despair. They begin to blame self and hide from others. The aggressor might begin crying, sleeping or just remain alone in a corner.

In some cases the aggressor does not show remorse and may be happy about the violence. What causes the cycle to begin is when interpersonal difficulties arise. When the interpersonal issues continue to add, the situation becomes different and tension begins to build; causing the cycle to start.

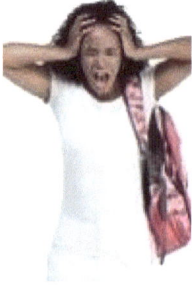

Positive talk and affirmation should be emphasized to decrease the chances of triggering another cycle of violence. The aggressor can engage in different activities like recreation and exercising to divert their mind. Mark the triggers of assault and avoid mentioning or accommodating them.

3.0 AGGRESSION AND VIOLENT PREDICTIVE FACTORS.

As assaultive behavior continues to become a major concern in healthcare, factors that precede violence have been discovered. The knowledge of these factors ensure the safety of the healthcare professionals as well as the patients and their families.

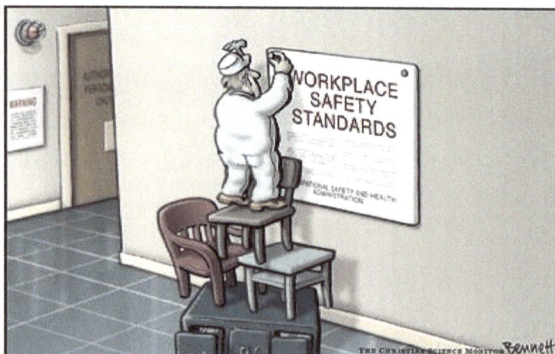

3.1 Demography and Personal History.

In the healthcare facilities, demography and personal history play a major role in providing information on the possibility of aggressive behavior. Chapman et al (2009, p. 476) mention that, *an individual who have shown threats of hostility and belong to a group or subculture that engages in violence could be a prospective violent person. Male patients are believed to have higher likelihood of becoming violent than women*.

Healthcare professionals take into consideration the history of the patient, healthcare worker or visitor.

AGGRESSIVE TENDENCIES IN THE PAST CAN BE IDENTIFIED AS A POSSIBILITY FOR AGGRESSION IN THE FUTURE.

Incidents of cruelty towards self and others are used to determine the possibility of aggression. The presence of men as the majority in aggressive behavior may not be necessarily correct in relation to violent behavior in healthcare.

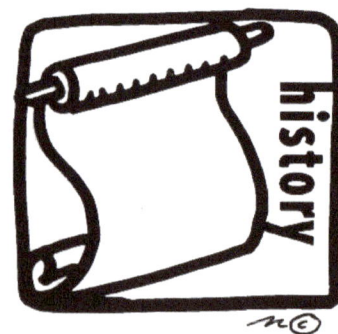

Young people tend to be involved in violence than older people. There is a correlation of low income earners, unemployed, low literacy levels being a contributive factor to violence.

Healthcare facilities report high cases of violence occur at night as opposed to the day. Aggressive people become violent towards the victim if the victim is alone and is female. When there is less surveillance from the hospital guards and visiting time for patients, violence tend to occur. When the aggressor sees that there is no security, they are likely to take the opportunity to exhibit violence.

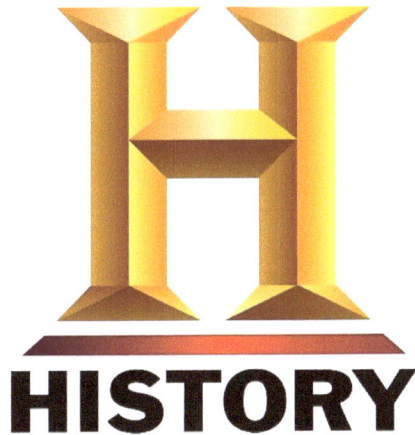

HISTORY

The frequency of assaultive behavior in a given population is used as a base line to predict violence. Use of rates of previous occurrence to predict possibilities is considered to be an actual factor.

3.2 Individual disorders, sickness and substance abuse factors.

❖ The individual may be having personal crisis where they lost control or power.
❖ Anxiety disorder is regarded as a ground for causing aggression and can predict violence.
❖ The aggressor may be on drugs.
❖ Delirium can cause violence if the patient has seizures, infection, and trauma or electrolyte imbalance (reversible).
❖ Brain injury, Dementia, excess alcohol and Alzheimer's disease can contribute to the development of aggressive behavior.
❖ Previous mental problems like paranoia, personality disorders, psychiatric illnesses or psychosis can predict violence.

Morrison et al (1998, p. 558) argue that attacks towards healthcare professionals are not abrupt. Patients and healthcare professionals who become assaultive can be identified before they become violent. Prior to becoming violent, the aggressor will experience increasing tension, issue threats and become stressed.

History of violence is one of the reliable factors for predicting violence.

Employment, literacy level, ethnicity and gender are weak factors for predicting violence.

Loss of trust for the physician, visitors, relatives and other healthcare professionals in the hospital can lead to wild suspicions that will inspire aggressive behavior. Provocation to cause violence is a situation that may eventually end up causing violence **(Belayachi et al, 2010, p. 27)**.

Individuals who are unable to tolerate stress can become assaultive. People with psychiatric disorders such as schizophrenia, depression and bipolar together with schizoaffective disorder are prone to becoming aggressive.

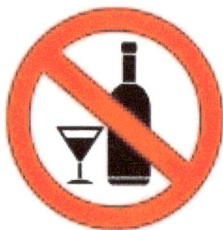

Substance abuse and excessive consumption of alcohol is a prominent contributor of violence in healthcare facilities. Patients with mental disorders and the psychotic consuming alcohol have a higher tendency of becoming aggressive than those who do not consume alcohol or abuse substances.

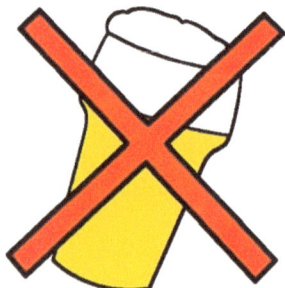

3.3 Situational Factors

Ferns (2006, p. 42) states that, situations that facilitate occurrence of violence can be used as a predictive factor. The availability of weapons such as knives, guns, sharp objects where the aggressor can access them could lead to aggressive behavior.

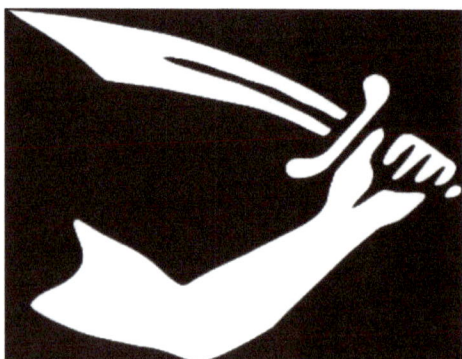

The presence of a person who stimulates the feeling of injustice, oppression as well as inequality can trigger abuse. When the person is forced to feel threatened and defenseless they become aggressive. Individuals who have experienced abuse from self or others in the past can quickly become aggressive if same condition is applied to the present.

If the person feels isolated from the rest of the people and is removed from their place of comfort without consent, they may not welcome the change and instead become aggressive. When something unexpected occurs, the event can stimulate anger which can eventually erupt into violence. There are prevailing circumstances that encourage violence such as overcrowding, favors towards others and uninformed rules.

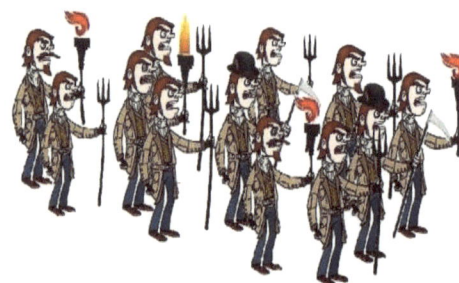

Healthcare facilities have been used as a holding place for detainees and people serving a jail term when the correctional institutions are crowded.

Sick prisoners are also taken to the hospital for treatment.

When in the hospital the detainees, can become aggressive to self, other patients, healthcare providers and other people within reach.

The Emergency room is usually a venue for assaultive behavior for the following reasons:

❖ Long waits could trigger violence

❖ Mental health patients' first contact before treatment.

❖ Patients with other diagnosis first contact

3.4 Actuarial and Clinical Predictive Factors

Prediction of aggressive behavior or violence has been given different approaches to include clinical actuarial and structured methods. Predicting violence has been seen as a very challenging task because assaultive behavior has occurred even in circumstances where no risk had been detected.

Actuarial methods of predicting violence take into considerations risk factors such as diagnosis, psychopathological condition, gender and age (statistical assessment).

Actuarial methods predicted violence if the same patient is exposed to same conditions in the future. As a result, the method does not recognize the judgment of the healthcare professional dealing with the current situation and is often used for admitted patients. Data collected on the specific patient is used to make the judgment if the person is likely to become aggressive.

Clinical methods of predicting violence have been used to predict overt behavior and consider factors such as psychopathology. Clinical methods are structured and assessment is done according to situation.

3.5 Broset Violence Registers

According to Abderhalden et al (2006, p. 17), prediction of assaultive behavior is possible during routine care. Healthcare professionals can forecast violence using the violence register on a short term basis.

Violence check list consist of six observations of the possible aggressive person. The observations include irritation, confusion, abusive and threatening words, and boisterousness, attacking animals and objects and physical threats. When the six observations are recorded, there is a higher probability of the person to become violent.

4.0 Conclusion

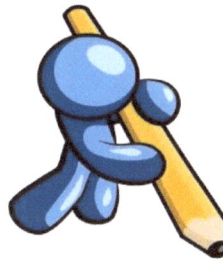

The assault cycle begins with a trigger when the behavior of a person changes and tension begins to build up. The next cycle is escalation phase where the body and verbal words reveal unmanageable anger. The next phase is crisis where the aggressive person acts violently. After the crisis the aggressor enters recovery phase when they begin calming down.

The final phase is post crisis phase where the assaultive person becomes remorseful. In an attempt to resolve issues the aggressor and victim can disagree leading to a trigger; hence the cycle begins again. This must be avoided. Ways of de-escalating violence should be exercised to prevent assaultive behavior.

Aggression and violent predictive factors include: Demographic (age, gender), history, disorders, sickness and use of substance, situational (prevailing circumstances), Actuarial, clinical, and Broset violence register predictive factors.

REFERENCES

Abderhalden, C. A., Needham, I., Dassen, T., Halfens, R., Haug, H. J., and Fischer, J. (2006) Predicting inpatient violence using an extended version of the Brøset-Violence - Checklist: instrument development and clinical application. *Bio Med Central Psychiatry*, 6, 17.

Adamowski, T., Piotrowski, P., Trizna, M., and Kiejna, A. (2009). Assessment of types and incidence of aggression among patients admitted due to aggressive behaviors, *Psychiatry Pol* 43(6), 739- 749.

Belayachi, J., **Berrechid,** K., **Amlaiky,** F., **Zekraoui, A.,** and **Abouqa**, R. (2010). Violence toward physicians in emergency departments of Morocco: prevalence, predictive factors, and psychological impact. JOURNAL OF OCCUPATIONAL MEDICINE AND TOXICOLOGY **5**, 27.

Chapman, R. Perry, L., Styles, I., and Combs, S. (2009). Predicting patient aggression against nurses in all hospital areas, British journal of Nursing, 18(8), 476-483.

Chou, K. R., Lu, R. B., and Chang, M. (2001). Assaultive behavior by psychiatric inpatient and its related factors. *Journal of Nursing Research*, 9 (15), 139- 151.

Ferns, T. (2006) Violence, aggression and physical assault in healthcare settings. *Nursing Standard,* 13, 42.

Ford, K., Byrt, R and James, D. (2010). Preventing and Reducing Aggression and Violence in Health and Social Care: A Holistic Approach. UK: M&K Update Ltd

Linsley, P. (2006). *Violence and Aggression in the Workplace: A Practical Guide for All Healthcare Staff.* Abingdon: Radcliffe Publishing.

Morrison, J. L., Lantos, J. D., Levinson, W. (1998). Aggression and Violence Directed Toward Physicians. *Journal of general Internal medicine*, 13(8), 556- 561.

Salmon, N., and Varela, R. (2007) *Learning to manage assaultive behavior.* New York: AMN Healthcare Services Inc.

CHAPTER FOUR

<u>OUTLINE</u>

1.0 **Introduction**

2.0 **Obtaining Patient History from a Patient with Violent behaviors**

   2.1 Identifying sources of information

   2.2 Preparing

   2.3 Eliminate triggers of aggressive behavior and use appropriate communication skills

   2.4 Gathering the information

   2.5 Identify common issues.

3.0 **Characteristics of Aggressive and Violent Patients and Victims**

   3.1 Emotional and behavioral characteristics

   3.2 Physical characteristics

   3.3 Personality characteristics

   3.4 Relationship with others

   3.5 Medical and substance use analysis

4.0   Conclusion

Crisis Prevention and Intervention in Healthcare

1.0 INTRODUCTION

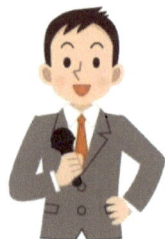

Healthcare professionals require the information of a patient with assaultive behavior to prevent and intervene in the event of crisis. This information is used in the implementation of appropriate preventive measures.

The traits of patients and victims of assaultive behavior should be recognized to assist the patient and the victim accordingly. This chapter will discuss how patient history with violent behaviors is obtained. It will also provide the characteristic of aggressive and violent patients and victims.

2.0   OBTAINING PATIENT HISTORY FROM A PATIENT WITH VIOLENT BEHAVIORS

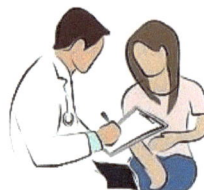

The history of an aggressive and violent patient can be difficult to obtain if there is no record. Hospital records should be handy when gathering information. The patient history enables the healthcare professionals give the most accurate intervention in a given situation.

2.1   Identifying Sources of Information.

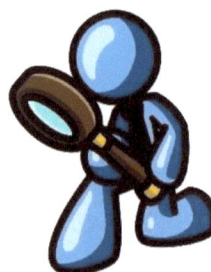

Obtaining information from patients with aggressive behaviors may be challenging because the aggressive patients are not usually willing to cooperate and disseminate negative information about themselves. *By the way, who would like to say something bad about themselves?*

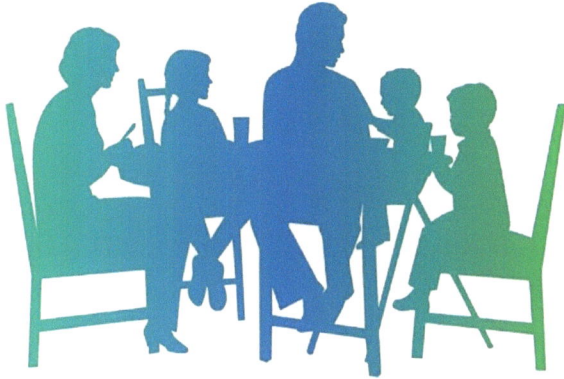

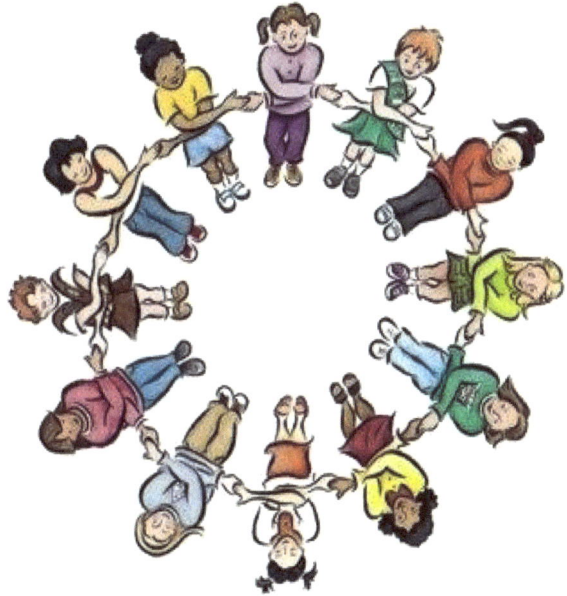

Friends of the violent patient can give additional information on behavior, for example, if they have been substance abusers. Some of the friends, family members, members of the public may have been victims of his assault.

The information can be obtained from family members, medical records, friends, and the police as well as healthcare workers. Some patients may be willing to provide information and be involved in the decision making and should be allowed.

Family members may be a good source of information on how current events happened and how past events occurred.

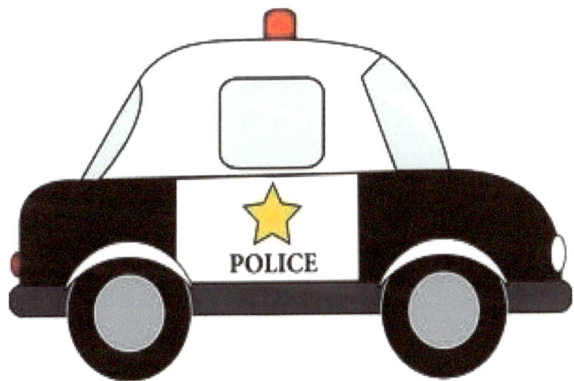

The police may have current and past history about criminal activities and arrests. The medical record is a reliable source of information (Dubin, 1993, p. 10).

2.2 Preparing.

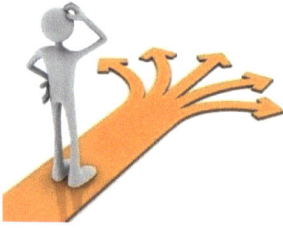

The history of a patient behavior and condition is very significant when it comes to making decisions on healthcare practice and should be conducted when the healthcare professional is ready.

Eichelman and Hartwig (1995, p. 84) suggest that, before attempting to gain the information from the violent patient, prepare self by clearing what is in the mind. If the records are available, the health care provider can view the last significant problem presented. Consider the available time for obtaining the information and if it is the correct timing.

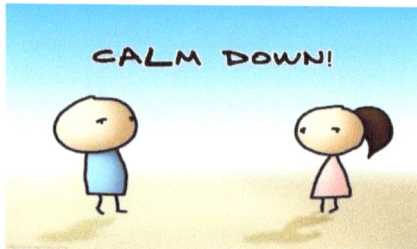

Develop a strategy to use in case the patient becomes violent. Handle the circumstances with confidence and calmness. Information should be sought after the patient and the healthcare professional are calm. Get ready for responses void of argument and heated disputes. The healthcare professional can acknowledge the upsetting situation the patient is experiencing and assure them of assisting them. Plan to de-escalate any possible trigger. Eliminate situations where the patient might feel confronted.

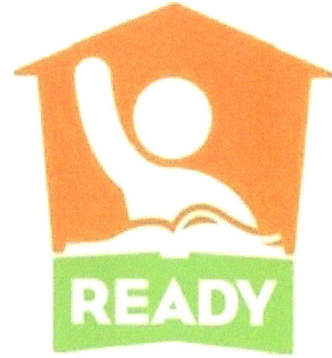

2.3 Eliminate triggers of aggressive behavior and use appropriate communication skills.

From observation made when the patient is aggressive, identify events that led to aggressiveness. These could include:

➢ frustration,
➢ intrusion to the patient's privacy
➢ anxiety, fear
➢ feeling threatened
➢ discomfort, and
➢ pain.

Manage their pain and avoid abrupt movement or noise. Avoid all the triggers that could lead to assault.

➢ They can be made comfortable by giving appropriate meals and adequate drinks.
➢ Keep away from rushing them to do something and inappropriate demands.
➢ Explain actions before you attend to them, give simple explanation and give them time to give an answer.
➢ Do not show when offended and evade criticizing the patient.

The healthcare professional can listen to the patient and avoid writing or getting distracted when what the aggressive/violent patient is saying is of relevance to them. If there is need to write, notify them and allow them to complete talking.

Take note of topics and activities that interest the patient and use them when necessary to call for their attention. Be a good listener and ask all relevant questions without offending the patient.

2.4   Gathering the Information

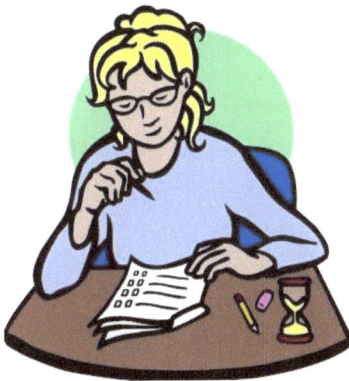

Obtaining data from patients may take different forms when the healthcare professional begins obtaining information. They may give single-word answers, may present themselves with a self-diagnosis and demand for medication, may need continuous reassurance, and may be angry or show tendencies of assaultive behavior.

Questions can be effective in gathering information if they are not addressing specific issues.

Polite steering of phrases can also help get information. Reassure the patient of confidentiality at all times. Avoid interrupting the patient when giving their first statement (Kanel 2012, p. 33).

An example is a patient that came into a mental health facility claiming that he was God. His delusion of grandiose was so strong that he was narrating his experience when he was being crucified, told of how he was so exhausted before Joseph of Arimathea came to help him carry the cross to Calvary.

As nurses obtained data during his admission, one of the questions was "Do you have problem with anger?". He was asked the question and immediately he burst out into a very loud and infectious laughter, laughing so hard and finally ended up asking the nurses "Does God have problem with anger?".

Information sought consists of demographics, which includes their age, gender and marital status. Find out if they have social support from friends, family or community.

Get details of their involvement in previous assaults, abuse of substance or alcohol and other sicknesses. Check and record physical traits that may imply involvement in aggressive behavior or crisis. Also, record verbal indicators that suggest the mental imbalance of the patient.

The healthcare professional should remain focused when questioning the patient, relatives, friends, other healthcare professionals, and police as well as when looking for relevant material. Concentrating and focusing on causes, concerns, and underlying issues that necessitated the patient's visit to the hospital is essential. It is very easy to be carried away by the patient's interesting history, thereby forgetting the relevant details.

The patient and their family or friends at times need reassurance and confirmation, which should be received well. Patient-tailored assessment gives the healthcare professionals ability to identify the needs of the patient and their anticipation.

Informed consent is vital

2.5   Identify Common Issues

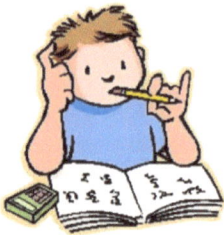

After conducting the search on the patient with aggressive and violent behavior, a record of the observations and information obtained should be documented.

This will be useful in the future, especially in the coordination of patient care. Information obtained will reveal what causes or triggers the violence, intervention that is given and the effectiveness.

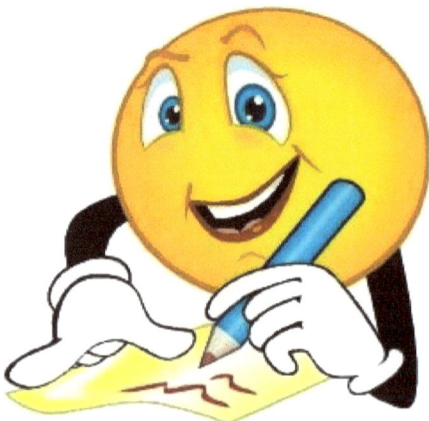

The information makes it possible to identify underlying issues that need to be addressed. Issues that are unique to the patient are identified. The information will give details of social history, medical history, family history, possible use of drugs and excessive use of alcohol.

3.0 CHARACTERISTICS OF AGGRESSIVE AND VIOLENT PATIENTS AND VICTIMS.

3.1 Emotional and Behavioral Characteristics.

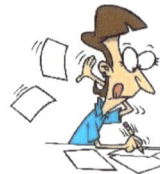

According to Shepherd (2001, p. 114), aggressive patients may show negative emotions such as anger, discontentment and anxiety. The patient is very irritable and unfriendly.

The assaultive patient could be frustrated from present, ongoing and future events they have no control over. The violent patients show signs of withdrawal if they have been abusing substance or alcohol.

Common behaviors that violent people have include
- constant desire to call for attention.
- agitation and restlessness.
- fear and emotional attachment in their conversation.
- augmented motor activity.
- disorderly, antisocial and disruptive.

Consequently, aggressive patients may become confused and become wild. The victim of emotional and behavioral assaults may feel devalued or dehumanized. Poor communication will cause hostility and misunderstanding.

3.2 Physical Characteristics.

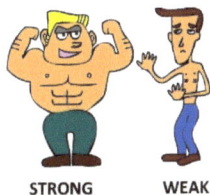

STRONG   WEAK

The violent patient can exhibit verbal or physical abuse towards self, healthcare professionals, relatives, non-relatives, animals or objects. Patients with assaultive behavior could be young adults in their early twenties or teenagers. Although majority of violent patients are young, there are elderly patients who become violent. Both men and women could possess assaultive behavior traits.

Although it is worth noting that majority are men, Women cannot be underestimated especially in the case of mental illnesses. Patients with violence might have had head injury and trauma. A violent patient may have a weapon, or objects that can inflict pain on others. Both fresh and old wounds may be seen on the violent person skin.

Aggressive patients use inappropriate physical contact to inflict harm on self and others. They use force to slap, beat, bite, spit and kick. The physical actions of a patient with assaultive behavior includes using unacceptable contact to create a situation that is uncomfortable and hostile. Victims of physical assault fear the aggressor.

3.3 Personality Characteristics.

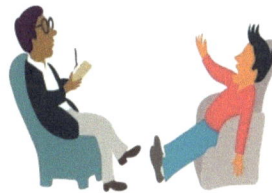

Aggressive patients have a low level of tolerance when they are frustrated. Violent patients at times reject criticism and want to be in control. They tend to blame others for faulty results that involve others or self. Patients with violent personality may engage in antisocial behavior, selfishness, careless driving and egocentricity.

Patients with low intellectual abilities can become violent when compared with the intelligent patients. Patients from low social and economic status tend become assaultive when compared with those from a high social status.

Violent patients may be comfortable with the assaultive behavior and live it as a lifestyle. In this case, the aggressive patient does not have remorse. Insults and aggressive behavior is used as a way of manipulating others.

As a result, the aggressive person becomes involved in breaking laws. Some patients with violence had been trained on violence as police or other law enforcement agents.

3.4   Relationship with others

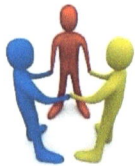

Aggressive patients tend to have poor relationships with the healthcare professional as well as the other patients. They may try to convince and take the other to an activity. They may not communicate effectively. Other patients who are calm tend to dissociate themselves from them.

The aggressive patient may want to intrude the personal or physical space of the healthcare professional, other patients, relatives or friends disturbing the existing peace. The patient may react negatively towards treatment, relatives or assistance.

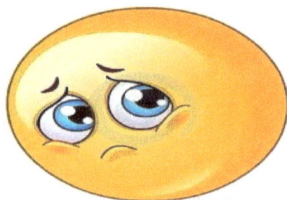

They may retaliate if they feel not treated right. Violent patients may perceive others as being in competition and fail to cooperate when granted help. The aggressive patient can provoke and tease patients, relatives, friends or healthcare professionals in the healthcare facility.

The healthcare professionals need to re-emphasize the rules of the unit and state the consequences of breaking those rules. It is paramount to remind the residents of the mental health unit that the staff are their friends and are working in the facility to ensure the improvement of their health status.

Since the presence of a poor relationship between the staff and the patient makes the potentially assaultive patient to become violent, the healthcare professional needs to ensure that adequate communication exists between the two parties and proper and therapeutic techniques are being utilized to ensure a very conducive environment.

3.5   Medical and Substance Use Traits

According to Tardiff (1999, p. 153), mentally ill patients are likely to become violent. Patient with bipolar disorder, depression and schizophrenia tend to engage in violence. Similarly, patients who abuse substance and alcohol are at times violent. Paranoid patients and those with hallucinations can become violent.

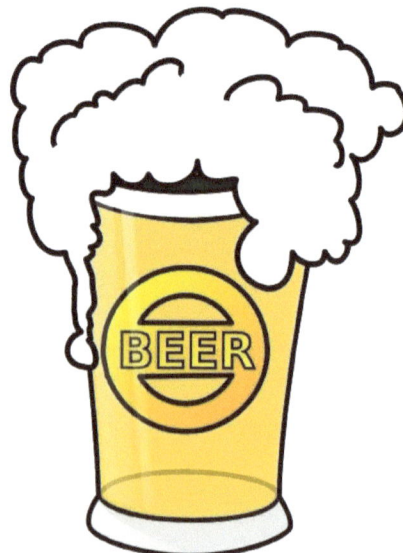

Violent patients may have depression, accompanied with hopelessness and suicidal tendencies. This occurs if treatment has not exerted remarkable improvement or if the patient does not adhere to the medication regimen.

The victim of violence becomes fearful and anxious after they experience assault. Their confidence and self-esteem is affected which could lead to a withdrawal from giving support or adequate healthcare to the patient. They attempt to change behavior and please the aggressive patient to avoid being victimized again.

The victims tend to withdraw and blame self for the aggressor's violence. They become tensed and guilty. They are terrified and may want to run away. In some cases, they may want to defend self by inflicting harm on the patient. Other victims feel ashamed because they were helpless and not able to change situation.

Healthcare professionals who have experienced violence may not want to continue working with the identified violent patients. If persuaded to work, they may demand that the patient is strictly cautioned about causing violence and verbal abuse. Injuries or bruises from the assault may cause indignity on the victim. (Blumenreich and Lewis, 1993, 22).

Healthcare professional victims who have encountered violent patients are pre-disposed to making medical errors and failing to satisfy patients' healthcare needs. Scared victims excuse themselves from working. The motivation to work for the same unit is negatively affected especially if the violent patient is not responding to treatment.

It is however very important to state that many healthcare professionals have been working for years in mental health units, and have never been assaulted or hurt by the patients because they have been applying the safety measures as outlined in this book.

4.0 Conclusion

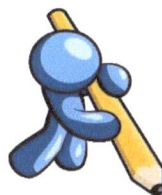

History of patients with aggressive and violent behavior can be obtained by identifying sources of information. Information can be obtained from the patient, relatives, friends, police, observation and medical records. Once the source is identified the healthcare professional can prepare self psychologically and physically.

Get rid of triggers of aggressive behavior and apply appropriate communication skills. Gather the information by focusing on relevant information and get the patient's consent. Identify common issues, and keep record.
Violent patients are characterized by negative emotions and behavior.

They may be physically aggressive and have personality traits of exhibiting violence. They have poor relationships with other people, may have mental illness or use drugs.

Victims of violence have fear, anger, blame self, are terrified and make effort to run away. Victims may have depression, low self-esteem and negative self-image. Some have injuries and tendencies of revenge. If not assisted, victims may hurt self or die from injuries.

REFERENCES

Blumenreich, P. and Lewis, S. (1993). *Management of the Violent Patient in the Treatment Setting.* New York: Routledge.

Dubin, W. R. (1993). *Clinician Safety.* American Psychiatric Association. Task Force on Clinician Safety.

Eichelman, B. S. and Hartwig, A. C. (1995). *Patient Violence & the Clinician.* Washington, DC: American Psychiatric Press.

Graham, A., Hamberger, L. K., and Burge, S. K. (1998). *Violence Issues for Health Care Educators and Providers.* Binghamton, NY: The Haworth Press.

Kanel, K. (2012). *A Guide to Crisis Intervention.* Belmont, CA: Congen Learning.

Kemshall, H. and Pritchard, J. (2000). *Good Practice in Working with Victims of Violence.*

Philadelphia, PA: Jessica Kingsley. McNeil, D. E., Hung, E. K., Cramer, R. J., Hall, S. E., Binder, R. L. (2011).An approach to   Evaluating Competence in Assessing and Managing Violent Risk. *Psychiatric Services,* 62 (1)

Shepherd, J. (2001). *Violence in Health Care: Understanding, Preventing and Surviving Violence: A Practical Guide for Health Professionals.* Oxford: OUP Oxford. Tardiff, K. (1996). *Concise Guide to Assessment and Management of Violent Patients, Second Edition.* Washington, DC: American Psychiatric Press.

CHAPTER FIVE

<u>OUTLINE</u>

1.0   Introduction

2.0   Verbal and Physical Maneuvers to Diffuse and Avoid Violent Behavior

    2.1   Non-verbal and verbal communication

    2.2   Tension de-escalation

    2.3   Anger de-escalation

    2.4   Substance abuse de-escalation

    2.5   Physical maneuvers

3.0   Strategies to Avoid Physical Harm

    3.1   Escape from behind chocking

    3.2   Stance and Front chocking

    3.3   Release of Arms

    3.4   Substance abuse de-escalation

    3.5   Patients with Weapons

4.0   Conclusion

Crisis Prevention and Intervention in Healthcare

1.0   INTRODUCTION

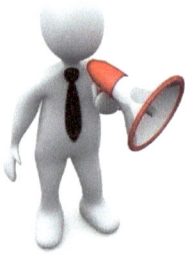

Putting off the chances of a assaultive incidents occurring could be life threatening. There is need to protect self from injuries that can cause decline in motivation and physical This chapter discusses physical maneuvers to diffuse and avoid violent behavior. It also explains strategies that can be used to avoid physical harm.

2.0   VERBAL AND PHYSICAL MANEUVERS TO DIFFUSE AND AVOID VIOLENT BEHAVIOR

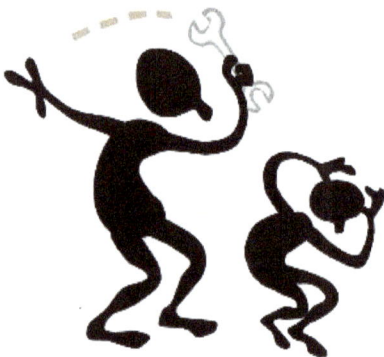

In managing assaultive behavior different ways of diffusing and de-escalating assaultive behavior are applied in an effort to prevent violence. De-escalating assaultive behaviors require the use of techniques when an incident is likely to occur to prevent assaults.

2.1   Non -verbal and Verbal Communication

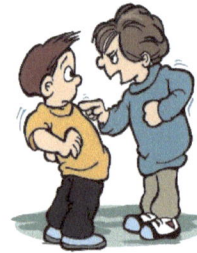

Clear and effective communication when dealing with the patient with aggressive patients should be adopted. When responding to patients, communicate verbally and write down the instructions that support conversation to rule out chances of misunderstanding.

Clear explanation at the beginning of the therapeutic relationship or when conducting a procedure helps the patient to know what to expect while helping the nurse obtain what they need. (Glick et al, 2008 p. 126).

When talking to the patient ask questions that are open ended and give adequate time to the patient to think and give a response. Respect the patient's space. When patients asks questions, explain in very simple but direct language. Avoid giving answers you are not sure. Use very simple words and short sentences when talking or responding.

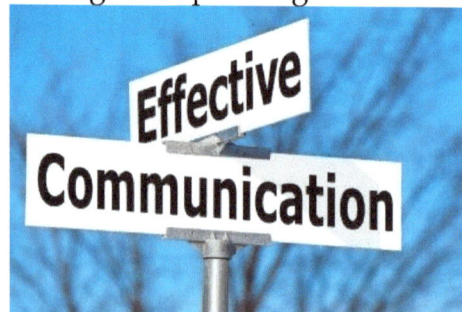

While the patient is conversing, allow them to vent their opinions. Direct eye contact, nodding of head, etc assures the patient that you are still interested in the conversation. Be neutral and avoid smiling unnecessarily which can be easily mistaken for mockery and stimulate anxiety. Keep away from touching the patient while talking.

Reaching out while talking to the aggressive person can be translated as a threat, even though it could be a habit that one is accustomed to when talking (Forester, 1997, p.42).

When they are yelling and talking in loud voice, do not scream to be heard. Remain calm until they take a breath, then talk to the aggressive person calmly. Be selective in responding to questions and attempt to answer the questions.

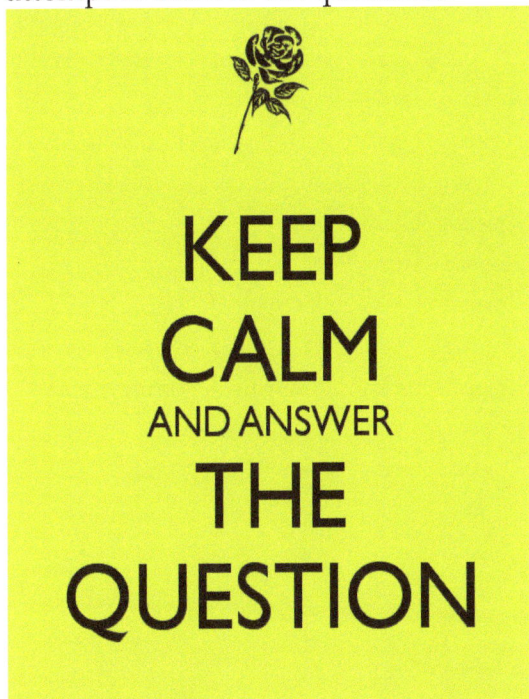

KEEP CALM AND ANSWER THE QUESTION

2.2 Tension De-escalation

Tension De-escalation is also called verbal de-escalation. In managing assaultive behavior the voice used should be polite, low tone and confident. Avoid talking when the patient is irritable.

In their study, Holmes et al (2013, p. 271) found out that

- the healthcare professional can manage behavior and avoid being inflexible.
- The body language can be controlled to avoid stimulating anxiety.
- A safe distance can be kept between the healthcare professional and the aggressive patient.
- Address the patient using their name and use own name.
- It is wise to obtain the patient's consent before administering medication or giving medical examination.
- Use clear words and attempt to clearly understand their response.
- Pay attention and listen carefully to every response they give.
- Be specific when asking and requesting for targeted answers.
- When conversing, avoid making promises. The healthcare professionals can express their desire to help.
- Assist the patient in expressing their thoughts and divert them from issues causing tension.

The situation should be assessed and de-escalating techniques employed before the patient progresses to becoming assaultive. Tension de-escalation can be achieved by attempting to solve the problem at the moment.

The healthcare professional can show empathy and give help if requested. Tension can be reduced by assuring the patient that they are not in danger and will not be hurt. Engaging the patient in a conversation or activity to divert their mind could help. Breathing exercises and relaxation can reduce tension.

2.3   Anger de-escalation

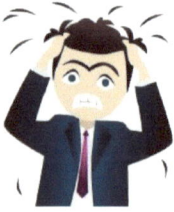

Duxbury and Whittington (2004, p. 476) affirm that when anger is not managed it can soar into violence. When the patient's anger is constantly increasing, it may be necessary to walk away and give the patient time to calm down. Let the patient vent and do not interrupt when they are angry. Be sincere when asked questions. After obtaining opportunities to have conversations, assure them of confidentiality and seek for their agreement.

In some cases it is wise to agree to differ in opinion. Refuse to give in to defensive positions and encourage the patient to cooperate with the assistance being offered. Healthcare professionals can keep quiet or walk away if there are chances of engaging in an argument.

Help the patient identify the underlying issues that are causing them to be angry. Healthcare professionals can facilitate boundaries that are practical and participate in implementing them. Avoid a situation that makes the patient sense interrogation.

- ❖ Be firm on the boundaries set and show respect.
- ❖ If verbally assaulted, remain calm and shun away from being defensive.
- ❖ Call for back up if caught up in a crisis. One can call for help or leave if de-escalation is not working.
- ❖ Hands should be visible so that it is easy to use them when needed. Putting hands in the pocket may be viewed as an attempt to take a weapon.
- ❖ Use hands appropriately without pointing or shaking fingers.

2.4   Substance Abuse De-escalation

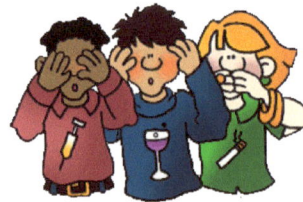

Assaultive patients who are under the influence of substances can be challenging to handle.

- ➤ Examine the area and space and ensure they are safe for the patient and the healthcare provider.
- ➤ When they engage in a conversation, seek to understand them and let them know what others feel.
- ➤ Keep away from the patients who have abused drugs and reduce the frequency of dealing with them.
- ➤ Remain proactive and be positive when it comes to assisting them.
- ➤ It may be impossible to agree, still arguments should not be accommodated.

2.5 Physical Maneuvers

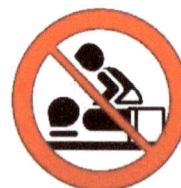

The healthcare professionals can acquire knowledge on how to deal with the assaultive behavior incidents in their area of specialization.

- ▪ Functional alarms can be installed at accessible positions in the hospital.

- The furniture can be designed such that there are no sharp ends and they cannot be used as a weapon.
- The layout of the hospital should be designed in a way that does not allow congestion and overcrowding of patients, visitors and healthcare professionals in a limited space.
- The rooms, corridors and facilities in the hospital should be ventilated and have enough lighting.

The healthcare professional should stand if the patient is standing and request the patients to sit down so that they sit down. There should be space between patient and the healthcare professional such that the patient cannot stretch their arm and touch the other person. The healthcare professional should not be directly in front of the patient but at an angle. This will enable the healthcare professional to escape in case of an attack.

3.0   STRATEGIES TO AVOID PHYSICAL HARM

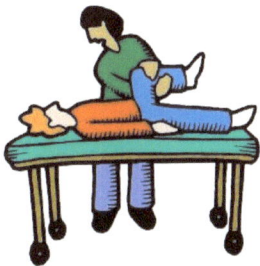

When developing strategies against physical harm take note of predictive factors and stay alert to take action when exposed to assaultive behavior.

When attempts to communicate, and de-escalate assaultive behavior are ineffective, STOP! Safety is a priority and help should be sought after by leaving, calling for back up and informing your supervisor. Physical means are used as the final remedy. Strategies to avoid physical harm entail finding practical ways to escape or protecting body from injury.

3.1   Escape from behind chocking.

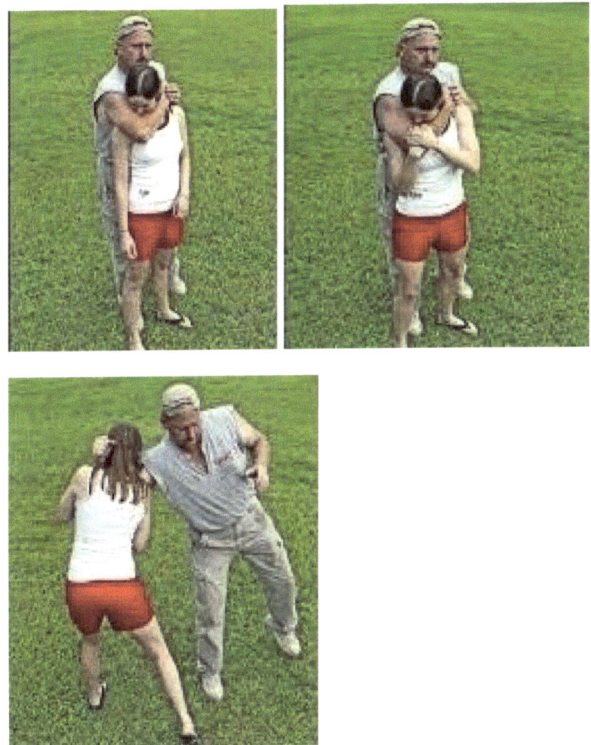

When attacked from behind gather confidence and remain calm and attempt to be in control. Raise both hands above the head. Then, twist to make the attacker loose their grip. While the hands are raised, twist towards the direction of the exit.

The legs should be twisted too to ease mobility. The healthcare professional that is attacked can twist hands downwards towards the completion of the twist to make the attacker arms unstable.

Upon release, move quickly towards the exit, and call the security for assistance right away. Release self by turning if the attacker has chocked from behind and ensure the hands are lifted to make the attacker loose balance and grip.

3.2   Stance and Front Chocking

According to Bowie (2009, p. 64), it is appropriate to keep the legs apart and wide, as well as leave the arms open when standing. There should be distance between the patient and healthcare professional. When the attacker is aiming at the head, keep hands crossed over the head for protection. Deflect towards the flow when the aggressor gives a blow. An aggressor who is kicking can be difficult to handle. The victim can protect self by turning body so that the kick hits the lateral area of the feet.

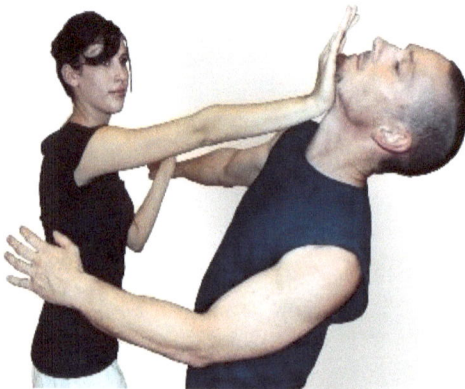

If the aggressor has attacked from the front, avoid backing up and continue being calm.

➢ Raise the hands higher than the head, a move which can confuse the attacker.

➢ A space between the shoulder and the neck is created when the hands are raised, causing the attacker to struggle with keeping the grip firm.

➢ Begin turning the feet towards the direction of the exit and then the body.

➢ While twisting the shoulders turn the hands downwards against the aggressor's hands; this will make the aggressive patient let go.

Protect the head from being hit when attacked, by covering with arms, boards or pillow (Bowie 2009, p. 64). Use the legs and feet to push away and prevent the aggressive patient from further attacking if one has fallen down. The arms of the healthcare professional can be twisted towards the attacker if their arms have been gripped by the aggressor. The face and throat should be protected always from being attacked. Master ways of avoiding the blows from reaching eyes and nose.

3.3 Release of Arms

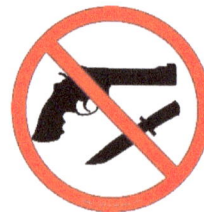

The patient can hold the healthcare professional arms tightly and refuse to let go. It is normal to pull or try to drag away, but this will not help. The most appropriate way to cause an aggressor to let go of the arm is by pushing the hand downward rapidly closest to the floor. Once the aggressor's grip of the hand becomes weak, quickly rush towards the escape route. After being free, keep off and call for help (Shepherd, 2001, p. 117).

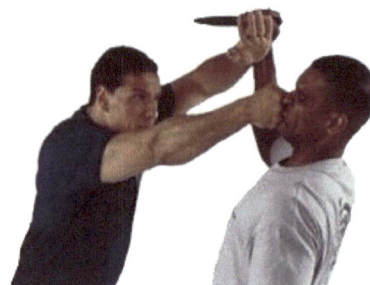

The healthcare workers can use certain facility accepted codes to define the kind of attack and when they need assistance. In case the patient is stronger than the victim, the victim can plead for mercy. Asking for mercy and crying can contribute to release, and can be used instead of yelling or becoming aggressive towards the attacker. But this is the last resort.

3.4   Punching, Biting and Pulling the Hair.

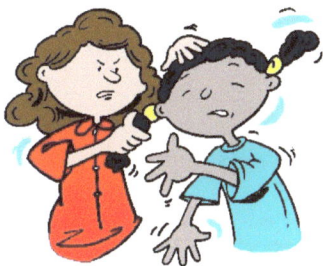

When the aggressor is punching, protect self by preventing them with an elevated shoulder together with the elbow.

Moreover, the elbow along with wrist can also be used to block punches. As the aggressor punches move towards their fist to destabilize them.

According to Duxbury (2000, p. 111)

- when the aggressor bites, avoid pulling. Bites can be eliminated safely by pushing inside the mouth for them to release
- When the hair is pulled, make an effort to get hold of the aggressor's hands and direct them towards the head.
- Change direction by bending to the front to make them lose balance. If the hair is pulled from the front, contain hair by pulling closer to the scalp and then twist to the front facing downwards.
- Hair that is pulled can be released by holding the aggressor's hands and pushing them down.

3.5   Patients With Weapons.

Some patients may be armed with guns, knives and objects that can cause injury. To avoid physical harm it necessary to CALL FOR HELP and stay away from them. If staying away is impossible. the healthcare professional should not reach out for the weapon. Being careful is emphasized. Stay clear of fighting back.

If the attacker has a sharp object and attempts to stab or hit, hold their wrists. Hold the weapon with the right hand and use the left hand to gauge their eyes. This exercise requires agility. Move to the attackers back and pull their jaw to the left while attempting to make the aggressor lie down. Let the head of the aggressor go between the healthcare professional's knees.

They can twist thumb and arm to take control of the weapon. If the aggressor is holding a weapon discuss with them and keep distance. Eyes should be kept on the aggressor. This attempt to defend self would be the last resort. Calling a code gray or green according to the hospital assault color, is the first thing to do.

When the aggressive patient is holding a gun at a distance, escape by running in wavy or zigzag line and duck if possible. Shouting and yelling to the attacker might not help. Avoid struggling to fight and try to prevent the aggressor from causing injury to the victim or the aggressor.

4.0 Conclusion

Diffusing violent behaviors involves using appropriate verbal and non-verbal language when communicating with a potentially violent person. It also involves listening, creating boundaries, and showing empathy. Violence can be diffused using techniques such as tension de-escalation, anger de-escalation and substance abuse de-escalation. De-escalation of violence is achieved by using correct tone and volume when speaking, avoiding confrontation, walking away, calling for help and letting the patient vent. Healthcare professionals show respect and remain calm when diffusing violence.

Physical maneuvers to diffuse and avoid violence entail installing alarms at accessible points, good lighting, avoid overcrowding and use furniture that cannot be exploited as a weapon in the healthcare facility. Keep distance and stay close to exit.

Strategies to avoid physical harm involve escaping and avoiding the aggressive person. One can free self if they are being chocked, held on the arm, bitten, punched or hair is pulled. One should avoid showing their back and standing close to the aggressive person.

REFERENCES

Bowie, V (2009). Coping with violence: A guide for the human services. USA: Whiting and Burch Ltd.

Duxbury, J. and Whittington, R. (2004). Causes and management of patient aggression and violence: staff and patient perspectives. *Journal of Advanced Nursing,* 50(5), 469- 478.

Duxbury, J. (2000). *Difficult Patients.* Oxford: Reed Educational and Professional Publishing Ltd.

Fauteux, K. (2011). Defusing Angry People: Practical Tools for Handling Bullying, Threats, and Violence. New Jersey: New Horizon Press.

Forester, S. (1997). *The A-Z of Community Mental Health Practice.* USA: Singular Publishing Group.

Glick, R. L.., Berlin, J. S., Fishkind, A., and Zeller, S. (2008). *Emergency Psychiatry: Principles and Practice.* Canada: Lippincott Williams and Wilkins.

Holmes, D., Rudge, T., and Perron, A. (2013). *(Re)Thinking Violence in Health Care Settings: A Critical Approach.* Burlington, USA: Ashgate Publishing, Ltd.

Leather, P. (1999). Work-Related Violence: Assessment and Intervention. New York, NY: Routledge.

Shepherd, J. (2001) *Violence in Health Care Understanding, Preventing and Surviving Violence: A Practical Guide for Health Professionals.* Oxford: Oxford University press.

Wykes, T. (1994). *Violence and health care professionals.* London: Chapman & Hall.

CHAPTER SIX

<u>OUTLINE</u>

1.0 Introduction

2.0 Least Restrictive Measures

2.1 Restraining techniques

2.2 Psychological restraint

2.3 Seclusion and Exclusion

2.4 Mechanical restraint and Four-point restraint

2.5 Restraining procedure

3.0 Appropriate Use of Medications as Chemical Restraints

3.1 Medication Categories
3.1.1 Butyrophenones
3.1.2 Benzodiazepines
3.1.3 Benzodiazepines and Butyrophenones

3.2 Atypical antipsychotics

3.3 Effects of chemical restraints

3.4 Administration of chemical restraints

3.5 Implications of chemical restrain

4.0 Conclusion

Crisis Prevention and Intervention in Healthcare

1.0 INTRODUCTION

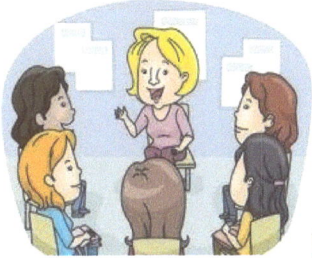

Restraining patients is a challenge because it has legal implications on the healthcare facility and the patient. The presence of a qualified healthcare professional is therefore considered necessary. Restraints prevent harm and can assist in the implementation of treatment.

Guidelines and policies on restraints are provided by regulatory bodies to ensure that the restraint is only carried out when necessary and does not cause danger to the patient. This chapter discusses restraining techniques and appropriate use of chemical restraints. Emphasis is placed on a restraint free environment.

2.0 Restraining Techniques

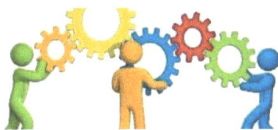

Agitated patients can be a threat to others and to self. The terms used in most mental health units are: Danger to Self (DTS) or Danger to others (DTO). Restraining entails restricting the arms, legs and strapping down the waist to reduce or contain mobility. Patients can be confined in the hospital willingly or unwillingly. Restraint prevents a patient from moving their head, body, arms or legs freely. Items used to facilitate medical examination such as bandage are not considered restraints.

a. Least Restrictive Measures

Measures to restrain patients with assaultive behavior are carefully selected because restriction or seclusion could lead to negative outcomes if inappropriately implemented. Therefore, recommended measures should be least restrictive and steered towards specific results.

Restraining techniques are recommended only when necessary. A patient can only be restrained following a physician's order. In certain cases, the registered nurse could start an emergency restrain, but must obtain a physician's order within few hours. Order includes the length of time the assaultive person should be restrained.

Healthcare professionals should be aware of the body alignment when implementing least restriction to avoid body injuries. The patient should be able to change movement and exercise joints a bit. Body circulation is important to enable the body to continue functioning as Ballard and Rockett (2009, p. 34) point out.

b. Psychological Restrain

Psychological restrain may precede chemical restrain and physical measures to restrain. Psychological restrain is given in the form of a program or a therapy. Activities are designed to meet the diverse situation of the assaultive behavior by withholding certain privileges. The privileges withdrawn do not include the basic needs. The patient being restrained will have access to shelter, clothing and food. Patients undergoing psychological restraint can interact with family, healthcare professionals and attorney. Psychological restraining is part of treatment which can be prescribed as a therapy.

c. Seclusion and Exclusion

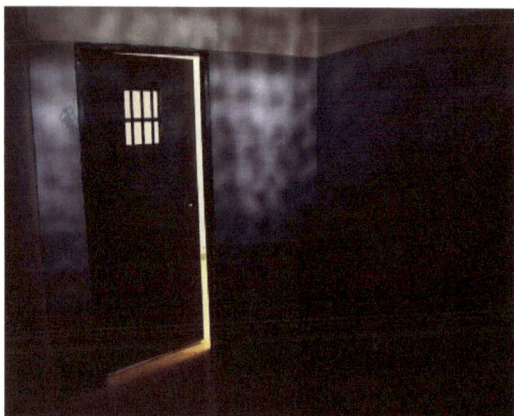

Seclusion implies that a patient is placed in a separate area from others where the room is locked. When a patient asks to have own room that is open, it is not seclusion. A patient is not in seclusion if they are locked in a room because there is a quarantine to prevent spread of disease. The room where an aggressive patient is secluded is not locked if the patient is a child. The room is often watched and secured. Safe and soft items are available for the aggressive patients to vent.

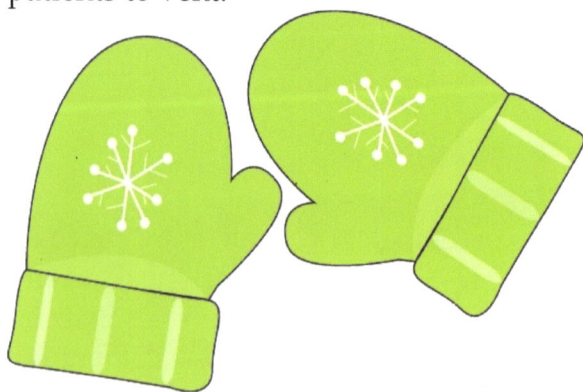

Mittens are applied to prevent pulling of IV lines, etc.

The objective of putting an aggressive patient in seclusion is not to cause harm, but to prevent the patient from becoming aggressive thereby reducing factors that encourage violence as Lewis and Ford (2000, p.34) discuss. Seclusion is given after the least restrictive policies have not been effective.

Exclusion takes place when a patient is moved from a one place to another restricted area. Patients with mental disorders who persistently do not cooperate with management intervention may be excluded from the other patients with mental disorders.

Exclusion is different from seclusion because in exclusion the room is not locked while in seclusion the room is locked.

Rooms for patients in exclusion are constantly monitored to ensure safety.

d. Mechanical restraint and Four-point restraint

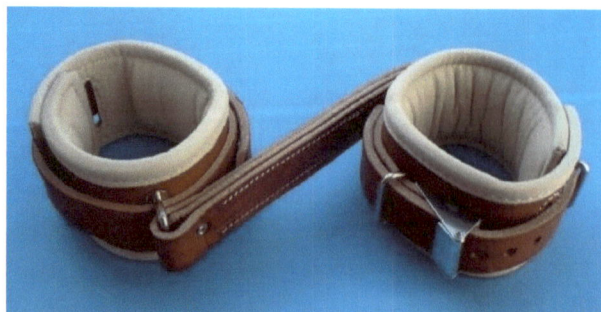

There are situations when the aggressive patient has acute violent behavior. The healthcare professional designs a mechanical restraint plan recognizing the imminent danger to self and others. The plan indicates how the restrain is to be carried out. Straps, mittens, wristlets, anklets, lockable buckles, vest strap, etc. are used. The patient may be allowed certain movements at specified intervals. Mechanical restrain should be applied carefully to avoid harm and removed safely (Park et al, 2007, p. 13).

When the de-escalating measures fail, measures could be put in place to reduce the chances of hurting the patient and healthcare professional while attempting to restrain them. Four-point restraints can be applied in the inpatient facility or the emergency room. The healthcare provider should ensure adequate documentation of continuous monitoring.

e. Restraining Procedure

Restraining a patient requires preparation to avoid incidents or injury. Healthcare providers with assaultive behavior management training should be prepared for emergencies and be willing to assist if required. Before attempting to restrain, obtain resources and the required number of people. Get the room ready before the patient is placed in seclusion or exclusion. Ask people by name to give a hand and inform them about the situation. Make a plan on how to approach the patient by assigning specific tasks to everyone. Reach the patient systematically and commit to play own part.

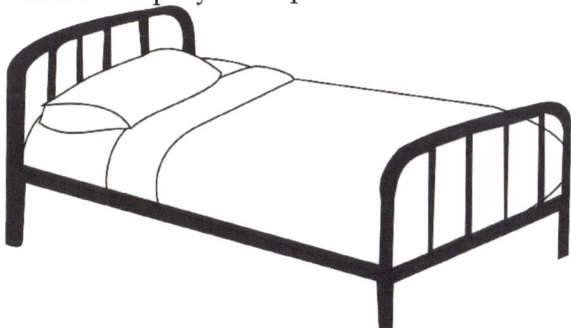

Appoint a leader who will give instructions when there is need to change the plan. The leader will assess the situation and make notes of the progress. Make an alternative plan incase events do not turn out as expected. The plan will entail a signal that there is success and a signal that there is failure. The leader will notify the team when efforts are fruitless and they should stop.

3.0 Appropriate Use of Medications As Chemical Restraints

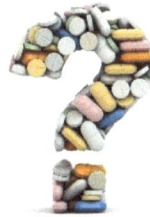

Chemical restraints are used to control behavior by administering medication. The medication is given according to individual's needs. The medication given to violent patients is short- term and is administered depending on the patient's history and circumstances. It is given on emergency to control behavior and to facilitate treatment (Mohr 2010, p. 5).

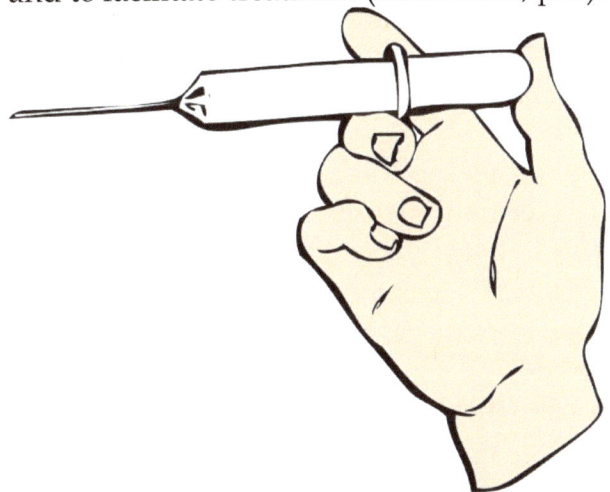

f. Medication Categories

Chlorpromazine is a medication that was used to sedate aggressive patients.

However, Chlorpromazine's usefulness has been exceeded by adverse effects on tolerance; hence its use has been discontinued. Butyrophenones have been prescribed as an effective and safe medication for use in containing violent patients. Butyrophenones have been successfully used together with benzodiazepines to restrain the assaultive behavior patient.

i. Butyrophenones

Dropridol and haloperidol are Butyrophenones, which are also Neuroleptics. Dropridol is appropriate for agitation which causes sedation. Dropridol is a first line medication. Haloperidol is a tranquilizer for calming patients with violence. The medication is given in the form of injection. Dropridol and haloperidol are safe to use for those with substance abuse or overdose, but will require monitoring. Butyrophenones are also known as typical antipsychotics.

ii. Benzodiazepines

Benzodiazepines in the form of lorazepam and midazolam can also be used to cause tranquilization effects. Lorazepam is considered the best because of its short half-life, rapidness, inactive metabolites and effectiveness. Midazolam effects take a shorter time than Lorazepam, but is fast in effect and safe. Benzodiazepines are specifically recommended for patients with intoxication. Assaultive patients can be given Benzodiazepines for control successfully.

iii. Benzodiazepines and Butyrophenones

A Combination of Benzodiazepines and Butyrophenones give superior effects than if used alone. One of the successful combinations is haloperidol and lorazepam.

g. Atypical antipsychotics

Risperidone, ziprasidone and olanzapine are in the category of atypical antipsychotics. The medication is a recent development that corrects the negative effects of extrapyramidal symptoms. The medications have improved outcomes when compared with Butyrophenones. Atypical antipsychotics are tolerable by different groups of patients. The medication is specifically effective on patients with mental disorders in the short-term treatment.

h. Effects of Chemical Restraints

Chemical restraints may have effects such as depression of respiration and will require monitoring and proper adherence to policies to ensure safety. The chemical restraint is prescribed by the physician. Assessment is done on the patient's response on vital body organs and body response to the treatment.

Healthcare professionals should follow the recommended dosage according to the age of the agitated patient. Medication on pregnant and lactating mothers should be avoided if possible. *Physical restraint* is not recommended for pregnant women because of injury to the spine when in the second and third trimester; hence *chemical restraints* are recommended. Neuroleptics should not be given to women who are pregnant or nursing.

Medication should be discontinued if it causes negative effects (allergy) on the patient. Patients with intoxication should not be given Neuroleptics, since it could cause seizures. Additional concern emerges since the medication could expose the fetus to abnormalities in development. Pregnant women are likely to develop respiratory issues. The fetus could have poor brain growth. Because there is no certainty if the chemical restrain could cause harm to the fetus, it is advisable to use minimal dosage.

i. Administrations of chemical restraints

The effect of chemical restraint is rapid and there seems to be reduced side effects. Giving the medication orally is preferred to intramuscular administration. Intramuscular administration is preferred if the patient does not cooperate and if there is imminent danger. Patients offered oral medication before intramuscular injection tend to trust the healthcare professionals which enable the delivery of efficient service.

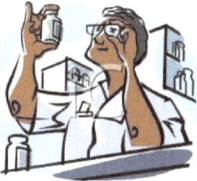

This is because the patient gains an internal form of control as opposed to external control from the healthcare professional. Dissolving formulas and oral concentrated are preferred to the tablets. Tablets are discouraged because patients can hide them in the mouth and fail to swallow. In mental health, it is called 'cheecking' medications.

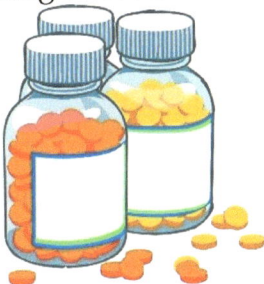

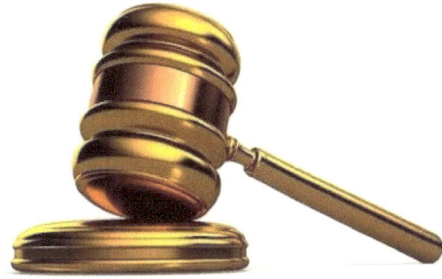

j. Implications of chemical restraint

Legal implications should be considered when a patient is restrained. Healthcare professionals would have to make professional judgment before choosing the chemical restraint because the patient has a right to and can make a complaint.

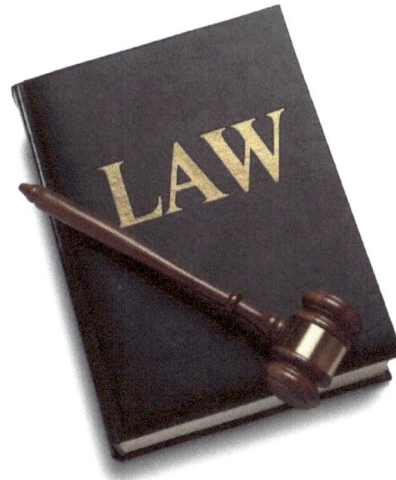

The healthcare professional should obtain an informed consent from the patient and explain the treatment if they are of sound mind. The patient can reject or accept medication for restrain if they understand the course of treatment. If the patient is incompetent and poses immediate danger, the healthcare professional can proceed with chemical restraints without consent.

A restrain free environment is emphasized to prevent the negative effects of restrain. Patients under restrain have been found to suffer injuries from falls, broken bones, impaired circulation, incontinence, social isolation and depression.

4.0 CONCLUSION

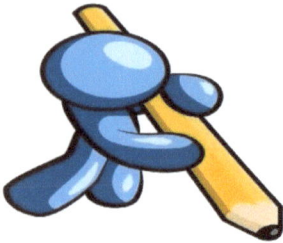

Restraining is done to prevent harm on patient and others. It sometimes enables healthcare professionals treat and control behavior of patient. Restraining techniques often implemented consist of least restrictive measures, psychological, seclusion and exclusion, mechanical and four-point restraint.

The strategies protect the rights of patients and are based on individual needs. Restraining is recommended and implemented by healthcare providers who monitor the progress and give recommendation. Restraints are administered and removed safely by trained healthcare professionals. Regulatory bodies recommend less restraining procedures, time limits and keeping of a record.

Chemical restraints are used if other restraining techniques prove futile. Medications that are used include: Benzodiazepines (lorazepam, midazolam), Butyrophenones (dropridol, haloperidol), and atypical antipsychotics (ziprasidone, risperidone, olanzapine).

The medications sedate the patient to control behavior. Although the chemical restraints are safe to use, they can cause effects such as depression, hyperthermia, mental conditions, and rigid muscles or affect vital organs; hence the patient should be monitored.

Chemical restraints are best administered in the form of dissolving formulas and oral concentrated or intramuscular or intravenous injection.

The healthcare professional should be aware of the legal implications to avoid pitfalls. A restrain free environment is suggested since it limits the number of injuries and other disadvantages associated with restraints.

REFERENCES

Ballard, B. and Rockett, J. (2009). *Restraint & Handling for Veterinary Technicians & Assistants*. United States: Delmar Cengage Learning.

Center for Ethics and Human Rights (2012). *Reduction of Patient Restraint and Seclusion in Health Care Settings*. Action Report.

Halles, R. and Frances, A. (2005) *Psychiatry Update: The American Psychiatric Association Annual Review*. United States: The American Psychiatric Association.

Johnson, M. (2010). Violence and restraint reduction efforts on inpatient psychiatric units. *Issues in Mental Health Nursing*, 31, 181–187.

Lewis, E., and Ford, J. (2000). *Hostile Ground: Defusing and Restraining Violent Behavior and Physical Assaults*. Paladin Press

Mion, L. (2008). Physical restraint in critical care settings. *Geriatric Nursing*, 29 (6), 421–423.

Mitzel, K., and Votolato, N. (2006). The use of intramuscular benzodiazepines and antipsychotic agents in the treatment of acute agitation or violence in the emergency department. *Journal of Emergency Medicine,* 31, (3),317-324.

Mohr, W. K. (2010). Restraints and the code of ethics: An uneasy fit. *Archives of Psychiatric Nursing,* 24(1), 3–14.

Park, M., Hsiao-Chen Tang, J., Adams, S., & Titler, M. (2007). Evidence-based guideline:
Changing the practice of physical restraint use in acute care. *Journal of Gerontological Nursing,* 33(2), 9–16.

Rund, D. A., Ewing, J., Tardiff, K. (1999). *Medical Management of the Violent Patient: Clinical Assessment and Therapy (Medical Psychiatry Series).* CRC Press.

CHAPTER SEVEN

<u>OUTLINE</u>

1.0   Introduction

2.0   Earthquake

3.0   Terrorism

4.0   Carbon Monoxide poisoning

5.0   Hurricane

6.0   Floods

7.0   Tornadoes

8.0   Tsunami

9.0   Volcanoes

10.0   Landslides

Crisis Prevention and Intervention
(Emergency Preparedness for Healthcare Facilities

1.0 INTRODUCTION

This chapter would discuss the emergency preparedness that hospital communities should observe during a certain suspected occurrence of a disaster. First, it is pertinent to note that disaster usually comes in all sizes and shapes; it can be either artificially created or natural. Suspected calamities are: the earthquake, landslide, hurricanes, floods, Tornadoes, terrorism, volcanoes, tsunami, weapon attack and lastly carbon Monoxide poisoning. It is advisable that since a hospital comprises of team work, the fight and preparedness here should also be initiated as a team.

Outside the hospital workers and patients, when people are anticipating an outbreak of any kind of disaster that may range from an earthquake, a disease, terrorism, and/or fire, hospitals are always on a high alert in view of intervention. This is necessary because if any of these outbreaks eventually occurs, those who become victims always require medical attention (Rout & Rout, 2002). Thus, putting in place a substantial medical system for attending any emergencies is congruent at such times.

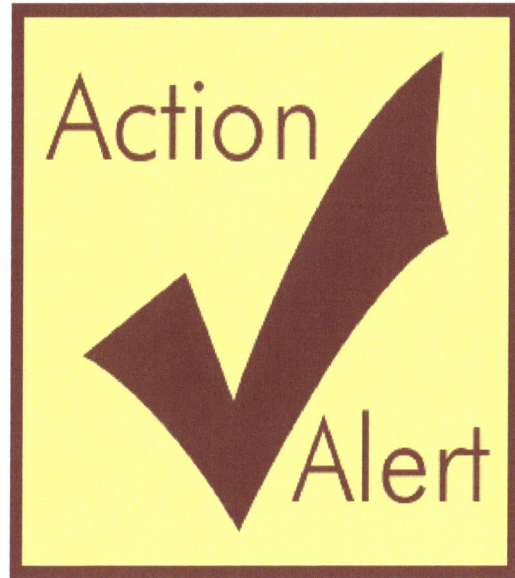

2.0 EARTHQUAKE

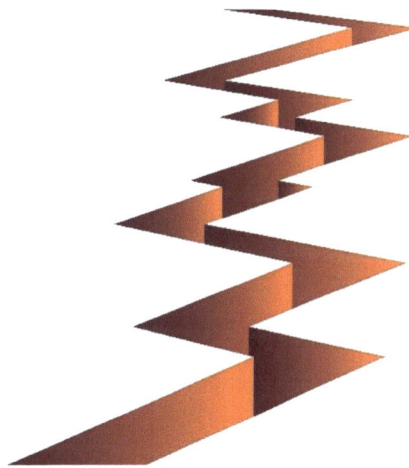

It is vital to raise concern over earthquake occurrence in the hospital. Earthquake is natural and often hard to identify the direction to which it is originating from without some machinery assistance.

It is advisable for the hospital management to be well equipped with several kits that can last over seventy-two hours after the occurrence of the real incidence. Some of the kits are the ponchos, radios for communication and networking, food rations and flashlights just to sample but a few.

It is also important for the hospital management to acknowledge the vitality of the emergency systems that will aid in notifications. Further, it is of awesome importance for the hospital to be safe-guarded with earthquake safety measures. Frames and foundations of the building should be reinforced to resist earthquake.

Whenever there is an earthquake, people should always drop, cover, and hold on. In real terms, this means that one should first look for a place to drop and cover him or herself when the earth starts trembling. This in effect reduces the chances of any person falling casualty of such natural disasters.

However, noting that the occurrence of such natural disasters requires that the inception of certain measures is substantial (Veenema, 2007). This means that if a certain area requires helping people survive an earthquake and thereafter reduce its health impacts, they must first of all prepare, come up with a plan, and practice.

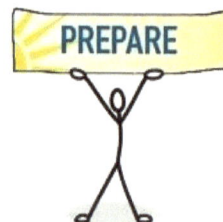

3.0 FIRE

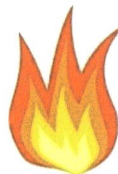

What starts as a simple spark can result to an uncontrollable fire in less than thirty seconds. Fire spreads very easily and requires just a few seconds to become risky and uncontrollable.

Nevertheless, emergency preparedness for fire with regard to hospital professionals is always significant (Reilly & Markenson, 2011). It comes to such a situation when hospitals' professionals seek to bring together the necessary equipment that can help reduce the consequences of a fire outbreak.

In whichever case, terrorism does not result into anything productive but rather diminishes any feeling of freedom and security within and outside the said territory. Take a look at the September 9/11 terrorist attacks; it is notable that both the American citizens and the outside world felt threatened security wise (Veenema, 2007).

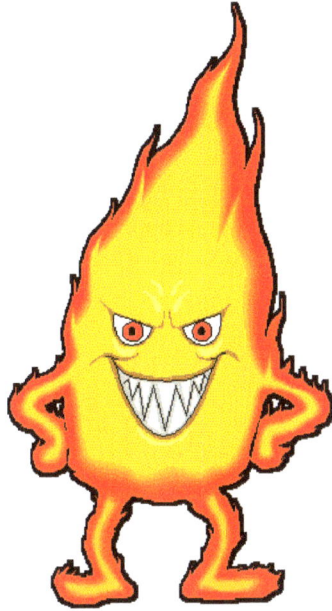

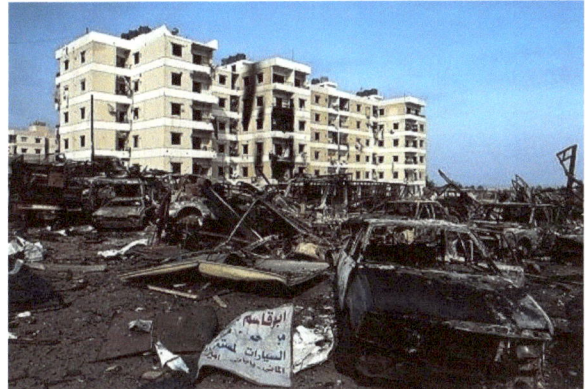

Under these circumstances, the level of readiness is very important as it helps determine the extent at which the hospital professionals will react to a fire outbreak.

In an event of fire, healthcare providers should have been prepared on the correct way to evacuate patients as the fire department tries to extinguish the fire.

4.0 TERRORISM

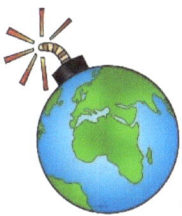

Some disasters may be natural while others are man-made. Terrorism is an example of a man-made disaster that may cause people loss of their lives and in other cases, loss, or destruction of their properties (Ciottone, 2006).

As a result, the government, with the support of other concerned organizations resolved to form such groups like the Local Emergency Planning Committees, which supports hospital professionals in combating terrorist attacks.

One way in which the hospital prepares for terrorist attacks is to be on the alert with heightened security system. Unlike before, people can no longer walk into the hospitals freely, everybody needs to be scanned for weapons, etc.

Exits should be properly labelled for easy exit. In addition, the alarm system should be in place and in good condition, which will help in getting outside help immediately.

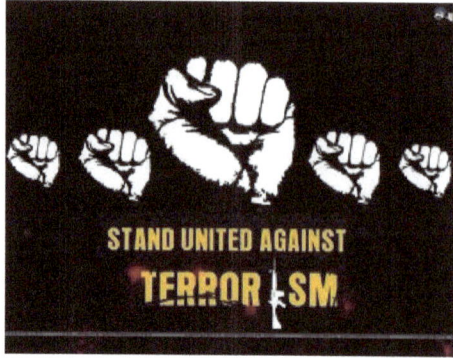

At times, terrorist activities may include holding innocent victimss hostage, shooting and wounding individuals, and/or releasing hazardous gases into an enclosed building.

Under these circumstances, the lives of many people are always at stake, a situation that calls for emergency preparedness in not only hospitals but also in security agencies (Rosdahl & Kowalski, 2008). In recent times, terrorist and other related criminal activities have skyrocketed and the available means of combating their consequences are being diversified. Hospital professionals equip themselves with emergency handling facilities such as masks and gloves if they are up against hazardous gases.

5.0 CARBON MONOXIDE POISONING

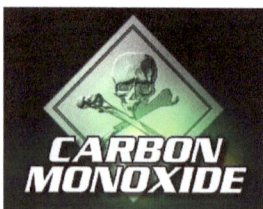

Carbon monoxide is simply a gas that is colorless and odorless but very poisonous when it reaches its maximum and can lead to a sudden death due to the body's lack of oxygen.

Carbon monoxide which emanates from motor vehicles, gas powered generators, fire, power washers, boats, charcoal grill, and other gas powered equipment can cause death when in sufficient supply within the ambient air (Ciottone, 2006).

The most at risk populations consist of the elderly, babies, infants, and people who suffer from chronic respiratory illnesses, anemia, and/or heart diseases (Landesman, 2005). In an event of carbon monoxide poisoning, hospital professionals should equip themselves with oxygen gas and resolve to consider carrying out hyperbaric oxygen therapy (HBO).

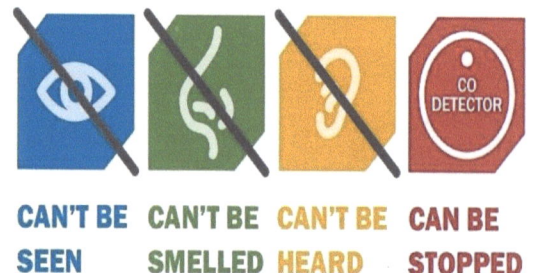

Oxygen administration is a substantial remedy against carbon monoxide poisoning mainly because it relieves the patient of hypoxemia as it helps supply the heart with adequate oxygen capable of pumping blood to the other parts of the body (Veenema, 2007).

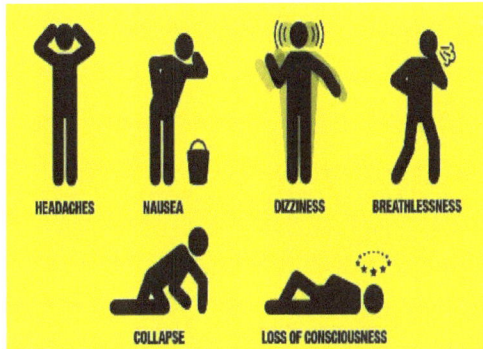

Healthcare providers should also show emergency preparedness in an event when a patient is brought in with Carbon Monoxide level above or between 25 and 30 percent.

In such circumstances, a patient may lose his or her life to cardiac complications, neurological impairment, and/or prolonged unconsciousness (Hogan & Burstein, 2007). Generally, when healthcare professionals carry out a hyperbaric oxygen therapy and diagnose a patient with severe acidosis, cardiac disease, or transient unconsciousness, they should always consider the situation as an emergency as the patient could die if immediate intervention is not proffered (Clements, 2009).

6.0 HURRICANE

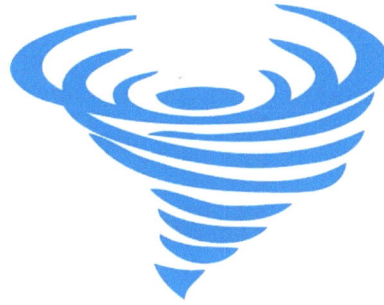

A Cyclone or a typhoon or other tropical storms could occur. Hospitals and healthcare professionals should at all times consider a hurricane to be a disaster that requires emergency attention and prepare for them majorly because they lead to the destruction of homes, industrial outlets, and social supplies such as water, electricity, and food (Rosdahl & Kowalski, 2008).

A hurricane is another disaster that needs thorough preparedness. For any hospitals to run effectively without worries of the severity of the hurricane, it is important that Back-up generators are rput in place to prevent black out condition.

In the event of a hurricane, strong winds blow. They tend to destroy power lines causing a total blackout, which leads to people living in particular area being cut off from the outside world, as they cannot watch the news or receive any supplies.

There could also be loss of lives as a hurricane destroys buildings, trapping those inside and making it hard for them to survive without the daily supplies.

With this respect, considering a hurricane to be a natural disaster that requires emergent attention is crucial for healthcare professionals as it can help save lives of the affected by providing them with the necessary medical attention capable of sustaining their lives (Landesman, 2005).

Hurricanes can trap patients and medical professionals in the facility without the ability of getting out, and that is if they are alive.

7.0 FLOODS

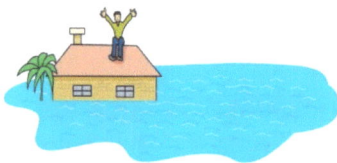

Another natural disaster is the flood. It is worthy to note that floods being a natural disaster calls for preparedness immediately when any sign is noted to avoid loss of life. Some of the preparedness process include:

- emergency teams being available so that they assist with evacuation .
- Plans are supposed to be in place for the relocation of the patients in the intensive care unit, those on hemodialysis and those who are in ventilators.
- safe routes should be improvised so the patients and other individuals can run to a nearby shelter, for instance a raised pucca house.
- Emergency kits should be accessible. The emergency kits must have; the torch, portable radio and spare battery. Fresh water stocks, candle, dry food and match boxes.
- Have grocery (polythene) bags, waterproof that can hold valuables and clothing

bamboo stick and umbrellas. Lastly, the first aid kit should have strong ropes that will assist in tying and manuals.

In relation to the community, healthcare professionals should prepare for floods. Floods cause diseases, infections, and other malicious ailments that cause deaths and loss of properties (Rosdahl & Kowalski, 2008).

Buildings collapse and structured centers fall apart when floods occur. Healthcare providers should prepare in case of a flood since they result in diseases such as cholera and infections such as typhoid.

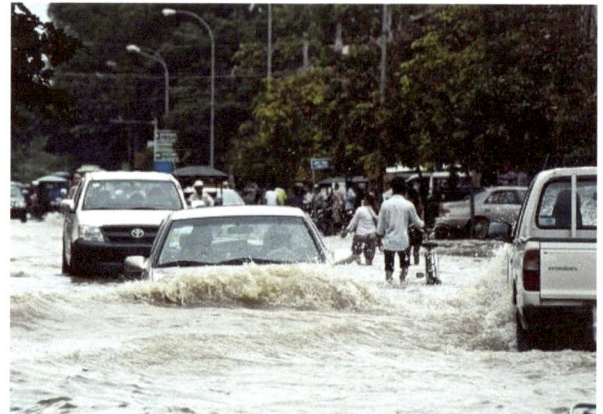

In tropical regions, floods cause other diseases like malaria since mosquitoes breed in such zones making it hard for the residents to survive in such conditions (Veenema, 2007).

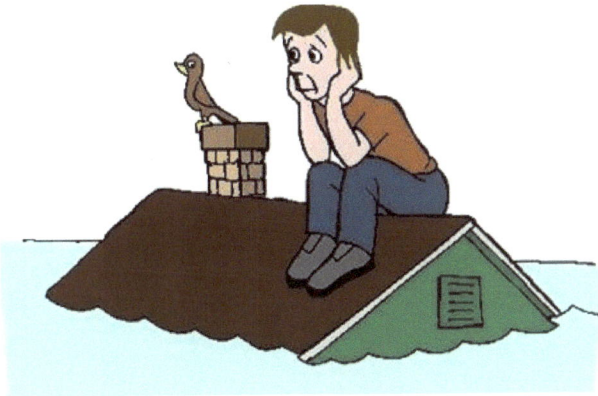

8.0 TORNADOES

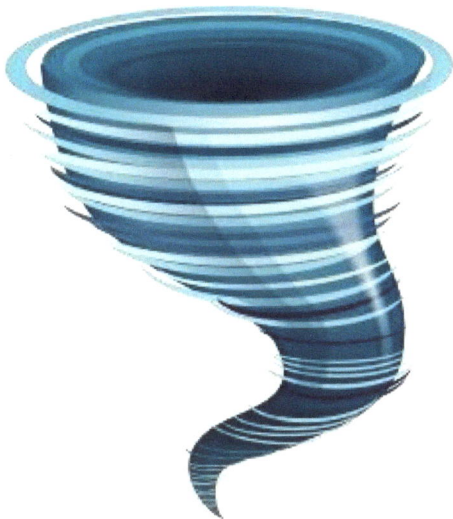

A tornado is another disaster that needs a hospital to be well prepared in any case it occurs. Since it is a violent wind, called whirlwinds and it usually crosses the land in a narrow path, it can cause death and so it needs correct measures to be put in place.

Here, the required preparedness is as follows:

+ the vulnerable parties like patients should be protected by every practical and feasible means available. Some of this practice are blinding and closing the windows.

+ Patients should be covered with blankets and nursing personnel are

supposed to move patients to the hallways.

+ All individuals should move to the interior, the hospital management should make the security available.

+ Any individual at the site that does not have security officers, should be designated as a spotter.

When people become aware of a possible occurrence of a tornado and immediately seek ways of evading it, the damage caused by such natural disasters can be greatly reduced.

Adhering to tornado warnings and implications can help save many lives as the set emergency evacuation and combating policies are always the best remedy for these disasters (Wolfson, Hendey, & Harwood-Nuss, 2010).

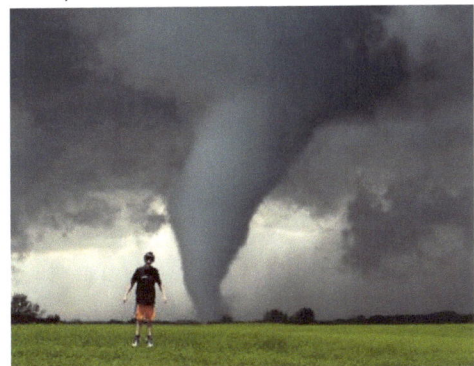

An ongoing tornado poses serious challenges and risks to people's lives as they carry with them heavily blown objects and risk killing people through falling or flying objects as the winds are always fast and strong. After a tornado, those wreckages that remain behind present additional risks to people's lives as they can result in risky injuries.

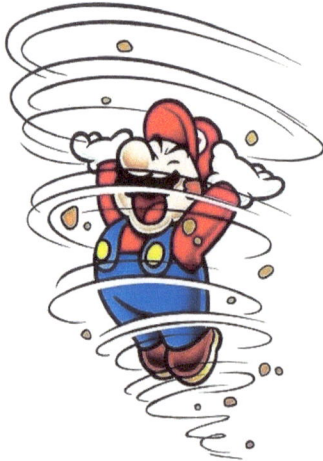

Nothing can be done in order to prevent the occurrence of a tornado but taking the necessary actions that can help combat the risks that a tornado poses is essential (Rosdahl & Kowalski, 2008). Just as in the case of other natural disasters, tornadoes break power lines, electrical systems, and gas lines and can cause huge explosions or electrocution.

Healthcare professionals should prepare for tornado occurrences since the challenges it poses are great in depth. Systemically, a wave of a tornado can leave hundreds of people dead and properties worth millions of dollars destroyed.

The rescue attempts of the tornado that took place in Marion, Illinois indicated that 50 percent of all the recorded injuries occurred during the rescue. People who walk among the debris may also sustain serious injuries as well as those entering damaged buildings (Trufanov, Rossodivita, & Guidotti, 2010).

When such a disaster occurs, people suffer many complications that require medical attention and therefore healthcare professionals should consider a tornado an emergency issue and resonate to set up an emergency preparedness platform (Reilly & Markenson, 2011). Medical buildings should be tornado proof.

9.0 TSUNAMI

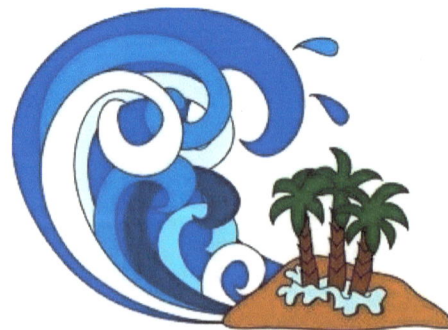

A tsunami is a long high sea wave caused by an earthquake, submarine landslide, or other disturbances. When a tsunami takes place, it is likely that many people will either suffer from multiple health issues or lose their lives in the process.

- Hospitals should carry out the pre-event preparedness, triage and patient evacuation.
- It is pertinent to carry out recognition of the hospital and secondary transfer, discharge where necessary and reduction of the admission procedures.
- It is pertinent for the hospital management to reinforce the medical system to be well trusted.

There is a clear indication that healthcare professionals should always be in preparation for a tsunami event since their expertise is crucial and can help reduce damage and save many lives (Wolfson, Hendey, & Harwood-Nuss, 2010).

Without a doubt, tsunamis lead to loss of shelter hence exposing the survivors to insects and heat among many other environmental risks (Rosdahl & Kowalski, 2008).

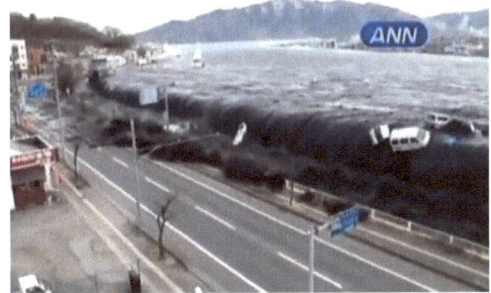

Majority of the deaths that occur during and after a tsunami are caused by many hazards such as drowning. Injuries result from people being thrown by water into debris, which include but not limited to houses, stationary items, and trees (Clements, 2009). During these moments, people may sustain injuries such as head injuries and broken limbs that commonly result from physical impacts when water washes the caught victims into debris.

10.0 VOLCANOES

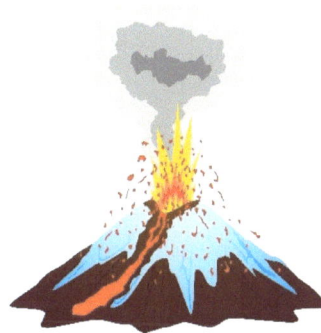

A volcano is a rupture in the crust of a planetary-mass object, such as Earth, that allows hot lava, volcanic ash, and gases to escape from a magma chamber below the surface. Earth's volcanoes occur because its crust is broken into 17 major, rigid tectonic plates that float on a hotter, softer layer in its mantle.

Volcanoes can end up producing flashfloods, toxic gases, ash, and fast moving flows of things like hot gases and other substances termed by geologists as pyroclastic flows (Rosdahl & Kowalski, 2008). A volcano eruption can also result to emission of hot water flashfloods and some debris otherwise referred to as lahars.

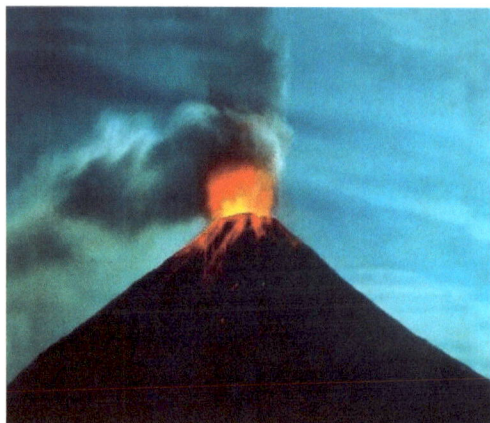

The emergency plan should include the following:

➢ hazardous zones should be identified and marked
➢ valuable property should be in register
➢ safe refuge zones should be identified so that hospital population can be evacuated if there are dangerous eruptions.
➢ evacuations routes should be identified,
➢ assembly point be marked, this will help those who are waiting for transportation to the next safe hospital to converge easily.
➢ Means of transport should be identified,
➢ presence of the alert procedures, still during evacuation, it is vital for health care personnel to improvise mobile treatment.

➢ Correct communications should be put in place. It is vital to establish a good system for updates.

11.0 LANDSLIDES

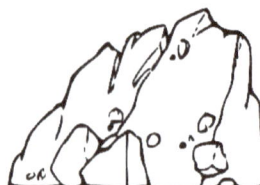

Landslides and/or mudslides occur when masses of earth parts, rocks, or debris fall down a slope making the neighboring parts sink together with the affected place.

Mudslides otherwise termed as debris flows are the most rampant types of fast moving landslides and tend to flow in specific channels (Clements, 2009). A landslide occurs when there is a disturbance within the natural stability of a given slope. Unlike man-made disasters, landslides can come along with earthquakes, volcanic eruptions, heavy droughts, and/or rains (Wolfson, Hendey, & Harwood-Nuss, 2010).

Since landslides result from other formations such as when water develops or accumulates rapidly on a ground causing a surge in water saturation on a rock, debris, or earth, it leads to an outbreak of diseases. (Rosdahl & Kowalski, 2008).

Landslides are so dangerous as even the hospital could be covered up in a landslide. If the hospital facility is not affected, it is the responsibility of the healthcare providers to give optimum assistance and intervention to the victims that has been brought to the hospital by the rescue teams.

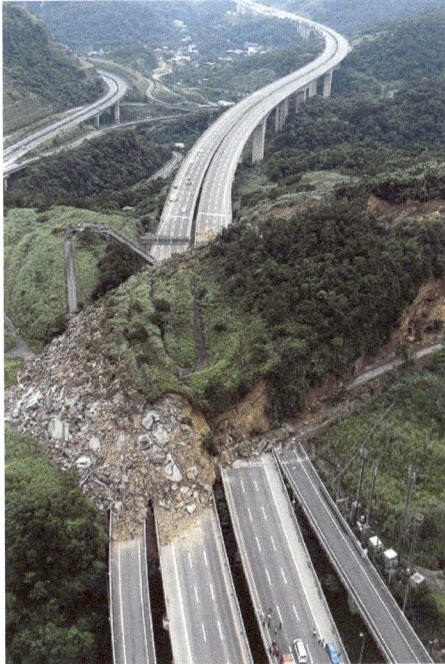

Further, it is pertinent for the hospital management to involve all the departments. By doing that, it will be possible to institute an effective team and collaboration process.

Another notable point is that, individuals should engage in not only practice but also training so that disaster management communication between the hospital and the community is effective.

Hence, everyone will have open minds and that when disaster strikes, they will be well prepared and will face it courageously and positively.

12.0 CONCLUSION

It is important for hospitals to revise their plans on how to cover additional types of disasters that have in one way or another been ignored. Here, a fact to put into consideration is to check if institutions are on the right track in their arrangement for the emergency preparedness.

REFERENCES

Ciottone, G. R. (2006). *Disaster medicine.* Philadelphia: Elsevier Mosby.

Clements, B. (2009). *Disasters and public health: Planning and response.* Amsterdam: Butterworth-Heinemann/Elsevier.

Hogan, D. E. & Burstein, J. L. (2007). *Disaster medicine.* Philadelphia: Wolters Kluwer.

Landesman, L. Y. (2005). *Public health management of disasters: The practice guide.* Washington, DC: American Public Health Association.

Reilly, M. J. & Markenson, D. S. (2011). *Health care emergency management: Principles and practice.* Sudbury, Mass: Jones and Bartlett Learning.

Rosdahl, C. B. & Kowalski, M. T. (2008). *Textbook of basic nursing.* Philadelphia: Lippincott Williams & Wilkins.

Rout, U. & Rout, J. K. (2002). *Stress management for primary health care professionals.* New York: Kluwer Academic/Plenum.

Trufanov, A., Rossodivita, A., & Guidotti, M. (2010). *Pandemics and bioterrorism: Transdisciplinary information sharing for decision-making against biological threats.* Amsterdam: IOS Press.

Veenema, T. G. (2007). *Disaster nursing and emergency preparedness: For chemical, biological, and radiological terrorism and other hazards.* New York: Springer Pub.

Wolfson, A. B., Hendey, G. W., & Harwood-Nuss, A. (2010). *Harwood-Nuss' clinical practice of emergency medicine.* Philadelphia, PA: Lippincott Williams & Wilkins.

www.ingramcontent.com/pod-product-compliance
Lightning Source LLC
Chambersburg PA
CBHW041723210326
41598CB00007B/761